I'll Carry the Fork!

RECOVERING A LIFE
AFTER BRAIN INJURY

by
Kara L. Swanson

Rising Star Press
Scotts Valley, California

Rising Star Press
Scotts Valley, California

"I Am A Rock," copyright © 1965 Paul Simon. Used by permission of the Publisher: Paul Simon Music.

Interior design, composition and copyediting by Joanne Shwed, Backspace Ink (www.backspaceink.com)

Illustrations and cover design by Mike Chrumka
Cover photo by Kim Scholtz

This book has been specially designed and typeset for easy readability.

Library of Congress Cataloging-in-Publication Data

Swanson, Kara L., 1965-
  I'll carry the fork! : recovering a life after brain injury / by
Kara L. Swanson.
    p.   cm.
    ISBN 0-933670-04-4 (trade paperback)
    1. Swanson, Kara L., 1965---Health.   2. Brain damage--Patients-
-United States Biography.   I. Title.
RC387.5.S93   1999
362.1'968'0092--dc21
[B]   99-33074
                                                                    CIP

To Mom and Dad With Love

Though now I follow better in your footsteps,
I'm still no closer to filling your shoes

Special Thanks to Special People

In this book I talk about many people whose support, expertise, caring and generosity were the building blocks for recovering my life. Several others made equally appreciated, critically important contributions before and after my injury. I want to give heartfelt thanks to:

Shirley Brothers and the extended Brothers/
    Edwards Family

Jan Sander

Bonnie Kissling, Kathleen Kubalak, Richard Rhode
    and the late Lynn Finkbeiner

Amy Baker Dennis, Ph.D.

Robert B. June and Sheila Thorp of Simkins &
    Simkins, PC

Christian Babini, Owner, World Gym, Shelby
    Township

Sheila Wyckstandt, Trainer/Nutrition Director,
    World Gym, Shelby Township: Ms. Michigan,
    1998 and national fitness competitor

R. Craig Hupp

Randall Kohn, DDS, Marie Wallace and Lisa
    Tatangelo of Quality Dental, Sterling Heights

Mike Chrumka

Kim Scholtz

Carl Goldman and Michole Nicholson,
    Rising Star Press

Contents

Foreword

The phone rang about 10 PM on January 31, 1996. The voice on the other end was familiar but it sounded far away, fragile, trembling. "This is Kara," the voice said. "I'm sorry to be calling you at home and so late but I was in a car accident today. (Tears now.) I'm all right, I'm going home but my car's been totaled ... I'm not sure why I'm calling you, oh ... my car ... I won't have a way to get to therapy this week. I'll call you."

My husband looked up and noticed my ashen expression as I walked back into the den. "Everything all right?"

"A client," I said. "She's been in a car accident. She said she's OK. I'm not so sure. She didn't sound OK, not at all like herself." I was surprised to find a tear rolling down my cheek.

I am a clinical psychologist. My practice is an interesting mixture of individuals, families, couples and groups dealing mostly with interpersonal issues, depression, anxiety and eating disorders. Early in my training as a psychotherapist, I was taught to guard against having an emotional response to, or a stake in, the outcome of my clients' lives. It is not considered professional, and is often considered to interfere with the therapy. Yet I have found that these responses are usually barometers of coming storms.

1

I had been working with Kara for about seven months. Shortly before her accident, we had uncovered her tendency to ignore danger signs and "red lights" warning her of potential problems in her relationships. Together we discovered that Kara believed she could endure pretty much anything, so avoiding disaster seemed unimportant. Kara was tough, resilient, a fighter determined never to be seen as a victim. She discarded the negative, denied it was happening. She was determined not to allow traumatic events in her life to define who she was. She was certain only the good things in her life would leave an enduring mark.

But the pain in her past kept catching her off guard. It was defining her in ways she didn't realize or could not acknowledge. We had been working at looking honestly at the impact of trauma on her and the way she responded to the world. Developing the ability to pay attention to the "red lights" and move out of the way of danger had been a critical goal of treatment. Ironically, someone else's failure to yield to a red light would soon lead to Kara's greatest challenge—and her greatest opportunity to do something she had always yearned to do.

The writer inside her, waiting for its season to blossom, was easy to sense. In fact, Kara was more able to reveal and process the painful parts of herself and her life on paper than in conversation. Early in treatment she brought me her journals. She wrote me letters, shared her poetry. The therapist in me found the writings useful pathways into her more secret self. The reader in me was mesmerized by her expressiveness, her poignancy, her humor and her style. She has a wonderful ability to laugh at herself, and to tell a story.

During this time she expressed her longing to eventually make her living as a writer. Kara's career in the catering industry, while challenging and successful, was a way to support herself, not part of her dreams. She was working on a novel when we met. However, she doubted if she had yet attained the necessary wisdom and experience to be a literary artist, and her busy schedule made writing The Great American Novel unlikely.

Her accident would remove the time obstacle, but create massive new obstacles. It would leave her with a brain injury. I had little idea what to expect.

We had been working on helping her follow her dreams before the accident, so I suggested she use this time away from work as an opportunity to write. But what she had done so easily in the past she now resisted. I was surprised: where was that driven client I had come to know?

The troubling answer was that for a while after the accident, her words and ideas just wouldn't come anymore. And she was afraid to reveal to either of us what she might have lost.

Kara and I talked about finding her a psychotherapist with expertise in head trauma. However, we had developed a trusting working relationship that she was unwilling to give up. We have since realized that there was another factor at work: she didn't want to be underestimated. I was the only person on the treatment team (other than her primary doctor) who knew her before the accident, and she believed I wouldn't allow her to settle for less than her best. We considered several options, then agreed to find our way together.

To be honest, I didn't want to give up the relationship either. Kara had been one of those clients who affected me profoundly. I had great interest in her recovery and in the way this woman was already redefining her life. I confided to Kara that I was involved in developing my expertise in other areas and would not be able to devote hours to studying the ins and outs of closed head injury. She decided to become the expert and teach me.

Early in my work as a psychologist, I learned a basic principle clearly expressed by Hugh Prather in his foreword to *Love is Letting Go of Fear* by Gerald G. Jampolsky, MD. "I can be of no real help to another unless I see that the two of us are in this together, that all of our differences are superficial and meaningless, and that only the countless ways we are alike has any importance at all." Kara and I would help each other redefine our roles and establish goals. I would learn about Kara's injury from Kara and the articles she shared with me.

Kara couldn't bring herself to work on her unfinished novel. It seemed irrelevant and she could no longer follow the plot lines of her own stories. But six months into her recovery, she began to write to me again. She started with stories about her accident, her frustrations, her treatment team, and her embarrassment at accepting help and support from friends. In the past, her writing had been a key to helping her find her way. It would be again.

She had begun to talk about this book and had already written stories about what she was experiencing. The words were coming more easily now, and her wit and style were gaining momentum. I began to push her. I assigned her chapters to write, helped her set deadlines, urged her to research the publishing process. She startled me with how quickly she had chapters ready to send to a publisher. No more foot dragging or lack of motivation. Before I had a chance to ask what the next step was, she was *on* the next step. She had begun to find her way, to recover a life.

I am often reminded that Kara is as much my teacher as I am hers. She has challenged me not to hide behind my professional persona, in much the way I challenge her to express her vulnerability, sadness and frustration. She pushes me to be honest about my emotional and intellectual responses and is learning that, at times, I withhold those responses to allow her own experience to emerge. I have become a more careful listener, and that has made me a better therapist, a better friend, a better wife and a better parent.

I'll Carry the Fork! takes you on Kara's journey. She details the events and challenges with great humor. That humor is a source of comfort, carrying her through the daily reminders of her limitations and losses. She has days when she cries and feels frightened and alone, others when she feels strong and victorious.

Ultimately, the book makes us see Kara as the complex woman she is. She will not be defined by her injury, her disabilities, her abilities, her success or her failure, but by all of these and so much more. Her story is one any of the sports teams she follows so enthusiastically would be proud of: coming back from a searing defeat, staging a stirring rally, and somehow pulling out a big win. May she touch your life as she has touched mine.

—Virginia (Ginger) Keena, MA, LLP

Catching the Bus

RED LIGHT BLUES

The curious thing about the auto accident that ended my life was that I lived through it. On January 31, 1996, Death sneaked through a red light disguised as a minivan going 50 miles an hour. 'Course, nobody told me that when they finished pulling me out of my car, they were putting me right on the bus.

That's what I call the process of recovering from traumatic brain injury: "getting on the bus." It's a good thing they strapped me down and fastened my head to a board. Had I understood even a little of the journey that had just begun, I would have hit the ground running!

I have always held the utmost respect for brave souls who face death with class and grace; who, with their last earthly breath, cite poetic verse on the meaning of life or seek to calm nearby witnesses from the awkwardness of impending demise. Luckily, I had no witnesses nearby. I had probably a second to sum up life as I'd known it. In the moment I thought I was about to die (to my vast surprise), I faced it with these courageous words of wisdom: "I'm fucked!" So much for class and grace.

7

I got pasted. To this day I have lost the morning of and the two days prior to my accident. I may have lost the third day also: wasn't that the day Publisher's Clearing House was supposed to show up at my front door after the Super Bowl? The sound of the crash of thousands of pounds of fusing metal was, I thought, unspectacular. Maybe I've watched too many movies. My first thought was how to get out of the car with the driver's side door lying in my lap.

They say the mind protects us from dealing with events too traumatic to process immediately. For whatever reason, I was a bit oblivious, entertaining myself with thoughts peculiar to the moment. I was happy I had just showered and shaved my legs. My mother's line (everybody's mother's line), "Always wear clean underwear in case you get into a car accident!" struck me as particularly funny. I was relieved my dogs weren't with me. I giggled at the thought that I had wanted to get the chip in my windshield fixed; the windshield now lay shattered all around me. I asked a woman at the scene to pass her cellular phone through what used to be my window so I could call my brother and tell him what had happened.

Perhaps I should have realized something was wrong when I didn't care that three young, handsome medics were cutting off my clothes and probing my naked body (I didn't even suck in my stomach!). Maybe I should have guessed that my brain had been squished when I could not think of where my brother worked or what his phone number was. Or when I allowed the woman from the emergency room to slide a bedpan under modest me without a second thought.

Seven or eight hours later, they released me with a gruesome headache, a new pair of scrub pants, ill-fitting crutches, and vivid colors on my body. I also left with the feeling that I was damned lucky. Blessed, if you will. Like I had walked right up to Death and tweaked him on the nose.

Witnesses at the scene called it a miracle that I survived. The police told me that if I hadn't been wearing my seat belt, the witnesses would have been treated to the sight of Kara flying out the passenger side window. Even as they pulled crumpled glass from some pretty incredible places on my body, there were no cuts and no broken bones, only doctors left shaking their heads in disbelief.

We celebrated my survival that night with pizza and painkillers (a favorite combination still). I told my bosses, who had stayed with me at the hospital and taken me home, that I would be back to work in a week, tops.

I wrote this book because the understanding of traumatic brain injury is *very limited* outside the medical community that specializes in it—much less among average "civilians." I left that hospital without a clue as to what a head injury was or what that diagnosis would soon imply. Every year, thousands of people join me and unknowingly bid farewell to the lives they had known. Whether the diagnosis is termed "traumatic brain injury," "closed head injury" or "severe concussion," many survivors are learning the tough lesson I learned: sometimes when your life ends, you don't actually die.

My doctor and my psychotherapist encouraged me to write this book. Not because my story is remarkable. Not because it's a tale of cosmic proportions. On the contrary, my story is unfortunately all too common. I wrote it because there are new faces on the bus every day. Faces of people who realize something is wrong with them, something they cannot yet understand. Faces that have no idea how lengthy and difficult the process of recovery is going to be. I wanted to write the book that I wish I could have read when I was first diagnosed with a brain injury.

Whether I have accomplished that or not, I honestly don't know. One of the residual problems from my injury is that I am largely incapable of tracking a story for long. This might be the first book ever written that the author hasn't really read.

I have attempted to address some of the potholes and barricades that I came upon—and often tripped over or fell into. I kept a journal, first to counter my short-term memory loss, then as a marker of progress and a sounding board for frustration and hope.

This is for everyone on the bus. It's about our hard-fought battle. It's for every survivor who fights that battle every day with courage and strength, frustration and wit, grief and confusion, begrudging acceptance and hopeful determination. It's for families who seek answers to questions they don't even know yet to ask. It's for friends and co-workers of survivors who find strangers hidden behind familiar faces.

It's also for the thousands of people committed to the prevention and treatment of brain injury. These medical communities, mental health practitioners and legal professionals offer care, protection and hope for survivors and their families. They provide counseling and legal guidance, and bring desperately needed resources to survivors who find themselves lost in a recovery they are often ill-equipped or ill-prepared to take on. Part of the proceeds from this book will help some of these people afford the tools they need to help rebuild lives that have been rocked to their foundation by the devastation of head trauma.

And finally, the book is for my personal support group. I came to think of them as TEAM KARA. I want this book to be a "thank you" to the doctors, therapists, attorneys, friends and family members who, when they realized I had gotten on the bus, climbed on board and sat right next to me. I am forever grateful.

Litter and Lingerie

MEETING THE MONSTER

February 2, 1996

I thought the dogs were just happy I'm home ... they've been sitting here in front of me all morning smiling and wagging their tails.

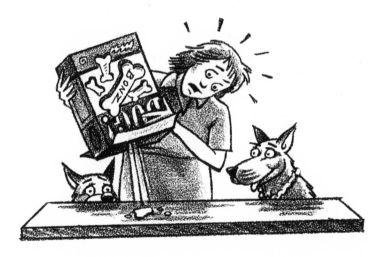

I felt truly loved until I found the empty 4-pound box of dog bones Diana bought them yesterday. No wonder they're smiling. I counted 13 used coffee filters in the garbage. Still warm ... what's up with that?

February 5, 1996

*I am sitting somewhere in the bleacher seats of my
mind.*

They say the first year of marriage is the most difficult.
You're learning how to live with a new person, what works
and what doesn't. You see facets of this person you have
never seen before and you realize some of the things you've
been doing for many years now need to be compromised.

Surviving a brain injury is like that, only the person
you're living with is you and the gown they let you wear on
the big day is open in the back and not quite as flattering.

Those first few days and weeks after the accident were an
introduction to symptoms I did not have the vocabulary to
communicate, the experience to understand, or the desire to
accept. There were things I noticed, sure. Peculiar things that
did not seem like me. But I looked back and recalled that I
had always been healthy and had always bounced back from
injury quickly. Unfortunately, I would soon find that I was
way out of my league. This was no sprained ankle.

My doctor, Sharon Cini, suspected a closed head injury
and confirmed her diagnosis two days later. When she told
me, I shrugged. I expected the pill or the shot, or even the
surgery, that would bring me right back to my normal life,
no worse for wear. When she started to describe a process
that might take weeks, months, or even longer, I simply
chose not to believe her. Nice woman, I thought, but certain
to err on the side of caution.

Evidence mounted, though. I couldn't remember from
one day to the next when people had called. I couldn't recall
when I'd last made a pot of fresh coffee—evidenced by those
13 used filters. My head hurt, continually, stubbornly and
brutally. I found my dogs outside and didn't know how long

they'd been there. I poured kitty litter in the washing machine instead of detergent. It was interesting to find my bras in the silverware holder.

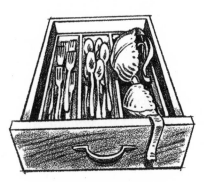

And I craved things. Weird things. Things I never really ate before the accident. White chocolate and lobster and pancakes and oatmeal. Corned beef hash and fried egg sandwiches. I ate plain, canned, boiled potatoes for three weeks straight at one stretch.

My friend Rita took me out about a week after my accident. Besides trips to the doctor, it was the first time since the crash I had been off the couch and out of my pajamas. As I walked, my legs seemed to have an agenda all their own. They were dipping and giving out and seemed totally oblivious to the concept called walking. Rita termed them "toddler legs."

I had already fallen twice in my home by that time, but I thought the lack of activity had simply weakened my legs. It seemed logical, after working countless 18-hour days, that the abrupt change in activity might affect them. I decided not to worry.

My family and friends didn't know anything about head injury. We didn't know how to interpret what we were seeing. Surely my problems sleeping were due to the medication. Surely my legs were just weak from being on the sofa for a week. I just needed more sleep, more soup, another day, another week. The problems would wear off like a bad hangover.

Most of the time I felt I was in slow motion. Everyone talked too fast. Words I wanted eluded me. I nodded and smiled through conversations that I had lost track of many sentences before. I didn't know enough to be scared. I figured I would just fake my way through everything until I was normal again.

My legs twitched and my feet were forever falling asleep. My left eyelid drooped and would open more slowly than its counterpart. I called my friend Dianne, whose mother is a surgical nurse. She relayed information on the tests I would soon be taking and suggested hopefully that maybe the medication was wreaking havoc with my body parts. Even after the initial diagnosis, I clung to that possibility.

Still, Dr. Cini threw me right into it. I saw her the day after the accident, a couple of days later, then once a week for several months. Thankfully, she had experience in head trauma and knew what to look for and how to proceed. I would learn later how many survivors go undiagnosed— sometimes for years.

She told me that we would have to wait and see, keeping tabs on the symptoms and noting them while my body worked to heal itself. She ordered tests and X-rays, scheduled appointments with specialists, and adjusted medications to eliminate the possibility that they were causing the memory and sleep problems. She wanted me to lie low for six weeks. I was incredulous. Work was piling up by the minute and I had absolutely no time for an extended leave. I gave in to two weeks and, for the next three months, allowed my absence from work to extend only one week at a time. It was my way of fighting, denying, refusing to accept the magnitude of my injuries.

I thought I would simply tough it out. If this big ol' bad-ass head injury realized I was not going to give in, it would soon concede defeat and leave.

Cane and Able

ACCEPTING THE DIAGNOSIS

March 4, 1996

I'm still tipping ... My legs still don't work right. They're usually fine if I keep walking forward but if I do that they'll find me somewhere in Canada by April. Tomorrow I'm going to see my work friends for the first time since the accident. Craig brought me over a cane. I don't want to fall in front of them.

March 12, 1996

I can't sing. Not that I ever could, mind you. But I can't follow the words! And my head won't stop, even for a day. Sometimes it's the "headache hood." It starts at the base of my neck and comes up the back of my head. Sometimes I'm wearing the "headache earmuffs." It goes right over my head and hurts until I can't hear. Last night I practiced dialing 911 with my eyes closed, just in case. This is, at times, simply miserable. Everyone has to get on with their lives, I suppose. It's no longer a simple act or a moment of crisis. Now it's turning into this whole new way of life. It's like the time after a funeral when everyone

stops bringing over bundt cakes. ... I feel really alone.
I want to return with them and leave this behind. I am over
it now and I want it to end, thank you.

March 23, 1996

I will never forget the first time I saw Mom after she
suffered her first stroke. She was lying in a hospital bed in
a hallway, her head tilted to the side. I looked at her, and in
her eyes was this fear I never imagined until today when I
looked in the mirror and saw those same silent screaming
eyes. I pressed my face up close to the mirror. I'm really
scared.

Evelyn Wood would have been proud. The first time I
decided to read a book after the accident, I made it down the
first page in seconds flat. I tried again, more slowly this
time. I read the first sentence and the next. And then, as if I
were reading in the back of a truck while driving over the
potholes of a Michigan springtime, I bounced around from
line to line. I read the words in the middle and a few here
and there, at the beginnings and ends of sentences. I closed
that book and simply launched it. Right through my kitchen.
With my cat running for cover and my dogs startled from
their sleep, I experienced the first of many snits that would
later be termed "bouts of inappropriate anger."

The tests didn't hurt at all. Well, maybe one, but I'll get to
that later. They were a little scary, sure. Any time you inject
dye into a person's brain to monitor its activity, I think a little sweaty-palmness is only natural. I was scheduled for a
CT scan of the brain, an MRI of the brain and one of the cervical spine. Because of the problems with my legs, I had a
lower extremity bilateral X-ray. I saw a neurologist and a
physiatrist (not a psychiatrist; that would come later).

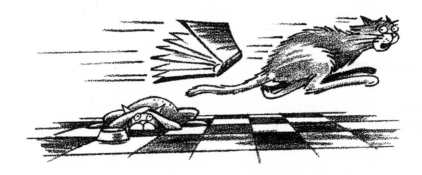

Results were coming back normal. There was no evidence of intercranial bleeding or structural damage.

I was seduced by the term "mild." Mild Closed Head Injury. Surely "mild" meant "soon back to normal." When, curiously, my doctors could not give me the actual "heal date" that I demanded, I simply created my own timetable for when I would return to my normal life. This they would later term "denial."

I did not respect the injury. I was beginning to believe that I had it, perhaps. But with the lingering bravado of youth I refused to entertain even the slightest notion that I would not recover quickly and completely. I started applying compensatory techniques before I even knew what they were. After coming out of the shower once with soap in my hair, and another time without washing it at all, I arranged the bottles and would open each cap when I went into the shower and close each one after using it. I started using Post-it notes for everything from who called to when the dogs were last out. I bought a whiteboard and started tracking my medications. Friends of mine, Diana and Marty, bought me a timer at the suggestion of MaryBeth, another of Dr. Cini's head injury survivors. I would take my "candy" (as friends euphemistically called the rainbow mix of pills I had to take) whenever the bell rang, like one of Pavlov's dogs.

The early answer was simplification. Trying to do all of the things I was able to do before my accident was not working. I could not talk on the phone and put dinner in the oven and open my mail and make coffee all at the same time anymore. I had to direct all the attention and focus I could muster toward one project at a time.

People in my life wanted progress almost as much as I did. They would call and I would tell them what little I was piecing together from my doctors. Part of the problem was that I was too stubborn to allow anyone to come in with me during my examinations. The information given to me in those examinations could have helped, had I been able to organize and remember it. Later, I brought lists of questions into my appointments and the doctors would jot down notes for me to take home. What I didn't understand or could not remember, I would simply fabricate, so I would be able to report some kind of ongoing progress. I was attempting to convince everyone, mostly myself, that anything considered "mild" could not be terribly serious.

Using a cane was a big step for me. We grow up thinking that canes represent the old, weak and frail. Perhaps I cushioned the blow with the belief that this would be temporary. I was falling a lot by now and I did not wish to risk that embarrassment in front of my staff. I was a catering manager and we were all used to seeing me throw a case of beer on my shoulder and run up three flights of stairs without a thought. All of a sudden, I was about to see these people in an arena that would spotlight my injury, and I was scared that they would see me as vulnerable, damaged, disabled.

But the cane provided me with the help I needed to not fall down and that was that. It was also a signal to people who might be driving or moving around me that I might not be able to react quickly if need be. It didn't mean *dis*-abled. On the contrary, it meant "now-better-abled," and that was the first of many important lessons I would gratefully learn.

It wasn't what people said, mind you. It was what they didn't say that scared me. I would sometimes catch them trading "those looks." I think we all wanted to believe that this kind of thing doesn't happen to people who are young and in the prime of their lives. Nobody wanted to hear out loud what each of us feared silently. We took potent injections of humor mixed with denial. Looking back, I don't know if it saved me or almost killed me.

I talk more about psychotherapy later in the book. But it's important to mention here that about a month into my recovery, I got very tired of hearing how "lucky" I was. This was not some vacation-gone-wrong that I would return from with horrific tales of adventure. From the moment I left that hospital, I heard slap-on-the-back choruses of "It could have been worse!" and "God, you were lucky!" Intellectually, I understood that. But emotionally, I did not feel very lucky.

Life sometimes seems so much easier if you compare yourself to others who have it worse than you. I knew I could have easily been more severely impaired, cognitively and physically. I could have died. But when you compare yourself to your old self, it's hard as hell. Late at night, I cried. When I thought about who I used to be and what I used to be able to do, I felt frightened and alone. Then the self-pity would kick in, and that made me feel ashamed.

Therapy became the place where I could begin the process of grieving for the life I had lost: something I sorely needed, and one of the hardest aspects of my recovery. The task was made more difficult by denial and the sickening feeling that I was somehow selfishly cursing Fate. I was detached from this person that didn't work right anymore. I didn't *like* this person. I looked at my legs with a strange curiosity as they ignored my commands and slopped and sputtered. I felt like an impostor. I feared that the longer this new person leased my body, the closer she came to owning it. And I was scared that people would forget, that *I* would forget, the person I was before. I knew I had to find her but I had no idea how or where to begin looking.

Coming to Terms

March 5, 1996

Tom was going to shovel my snow after work so I thought I would beat him to it. I fell twice trying to heave that stuff. People were driving by. When I fell, I started doing snow-angels so they'd think I meant to be there.

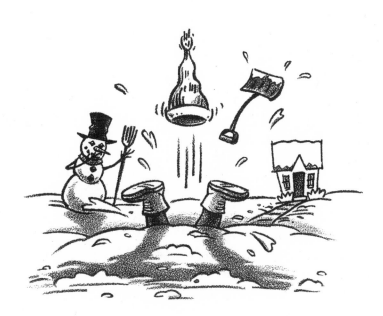

April 6, 1996

Cindy took me to U of M's medical library. We ran copies of everything we could find on head injury. Seems like you're either in a coma or anything goes. Not very comforting.

April 8, 1996

I can't juggle anymore.

I no longer had "toddler legs"; I was experiencing lower extremity, bilateral weakness. The back of my head wasn't just sore; I had point tenderness on the right rear crown. My headaches were no longer above my right eye; they were situated in the region of the right frontal lobe. My gait was ataxic, and my feet had sustained damage to the proprioceptive and protective sense functions.

Not bad, eh? Learning the vocabulary and researching the injury gave me a sense that I was leveling the playing field a bit. The more I knew and the more I understood, the more I was beginning to turn on the night light and unmask the monster.

I didn't just learn terms that first April. I started a series of physical, occupational and speech therapies that would provide me with invaluable information regarding my recovery.

I will admit I was a bitch at times. Quite frankly, I didn't like what any of my new therapists had to say. That first day they wanted to put me in a wheelchair because I was all over the place, tipping and dipping and losing my balance. I had a colorful response to that suggestion. They immediately arranged for me to have Carolyn, their most experienced therapist in balance retraining, take over my case.

Three hours a day, three days a week, for the next six weeks, I went through tests and tasks and trials and exercises. In physical therapy, we focused on trying to "find my center." We were trying to get my brain to recognize how to hold me still and upright.

It's hard to relearn balance when you have no idea how you learned it in the first place. I actually watched my friends' toddlers; they seemed to have more strategies for balancing than I did.

An important development came when tests revealed I would fall when my head tilted back a certain degree. Carolyn explained that my "clapper" was gone: normal people have a bell inside their brains that kicks in and tells them to catch themselves before they fall. Mine no longer worked. By stooping forward slightly and working to eliminate spontaneous reactions, I was able to greatly reduce the number of times I fell.

Progress was almost undetectable. Often we would just sit between the parallel bars, me strapped to Carolyn and surrounded by chairs. She would hold my knees and I would try to steady myself sitting on a huge ball. Or I would walk back and forth, holding the bars at first, trying to safely turn my head from side to side. In the beginning, spontaneous movement of my head would send me reeling. Between the bars, I gradually restored my ability to step over obstacles and turn to address someone who might call my name. Simple stuff. Things I had taken for granted. These were the slow, plodding steps and the minuscule progress that earmarked my early therapy.

Because balance dysfunction was the most pronounced and troublesome of my physical problems, other areas had been neglected. The strength in my hands was notably uneven and my fingers were clumsy. There was tendinitis in my right shoulder. I had lost certain tones in my right ear, and the muscles in my neck and shoulders were tight and rigid. After four months of inactivity, I was out of shape. I did exercises to increase my strength and coordination, and I underwent ultrasound therapy to regain mobility.

I was found to have 13 higher learning impairments: some mild, some moderate, a few considered severe. I learned that my tracking system was damaged. I did not have the attention and concentration abilities to stay in a conversation or follow a story for long. My speech therapist, Rhonda, would ask questions and direct me through tasks, and I would be looking at the pictures of her Dalmatians tacked above her desk. Rhonda and my other two therapists had the wonderful gift of feeding my confidence and preserving my integrity. Here I was playing with blocks and putting simple puzzles together—*kid stuff*—yet they made me feel very comfortable. They sensed whenever I was close to throwing those damn blocks and were able to calm me, divert me and inspire me to keep at it. Their patience was important as my journey through therapy continued to reveal deficits.

My ability to multitask was impaired. If I tried to boil the water for pasta and brown the meat for the sauce and chop the vegetables for the salad, I would end up with overcooked spaghetti, burned meat, vegetables on the floor, bowls flying through the kitchen, and me cursing a blue streak. I had to work on each item separately, without anything else out of the refrigerator or on the counter to distract me.

If I was standing in the middle of a room, I couldn't stay balanced and talk at the same time. A friend of mine once reached out to catch me, steadied my shoulders and asked, "Kara, do you realize you're swaying?" After that, I stood with my back to walls and hung on to furniture so I could concentrate; or I just sat down so I could have a conversation without fearing I'd fall.

Occupational therapy was supposed to be geared toward assessing my ability to return to work. When my occupational therapist, Donna, canceled some of our sessions so I could spend the time in physical therapy, I started to understand that returning to work took a back seat to safety. In the short time I spent with her, though, she made a significant contribution, uncovering a problem that contributed to my dysfunctional balance and uncoordinated gait.

When you step on the summer cement barefoot, or accidentally touch a hot stove, your brain reacts with lightning-quick speed to send messages that tell you to move. In my case, the protective sense in my feet had suffered a 94 percent loss and would not respond quickly enough to keep me out of danger. I also did not know exactly what my feet were doing if I didn't watch them. When I'd stand up or begin to walk, I had to check to make sure they were doing what they were supposed to do.

All of my therapists preached safety and caution. Safety and caution. Safety and caution. *Blah, blah, blah.* I often thought they had probably been crossing guards in another life. They instructed me to wear safe, supportive shoes. They timed my steps-per-minute to ensure that I could cross a street without putting myself in danger. And they made me repeatedly practice transfers from sitting to standing, on uneven surfaces, and from turns to stairs.

They encouraged my progress and, more importantly, my determination. However, they mentioned "windows of recovery" that often narrowed after three to six months (I didn't even get into therapy until three months after the accident), and spoke of the likelihood that even after a year I might see little improvement, if any at all.

I wouldn't even consider a year. I was busy preparing myself for basketball in August. Each season our high school hosts a scrimmage between the new varsity squad and a collection of alumni dating back to the class of 1973. I had not missed that game in 13 years and was *righteously determined* to make it onto that court. I told my therapists of my plan and their part in it. They were to "fix" me and do it soon. It had already been 6 months. That was plenty.

Instead, they took my cane and threatened me with a walker after I refused the wheelchair. I bartered down to crutches and they put me on a tether that friends would be instructed to hold when I was walking with them. In short, I was on a leash. My friends loved it! They would call and ask me if I wanted them to "take me for a walk." I'm sure my dogs enjoyed the irony.

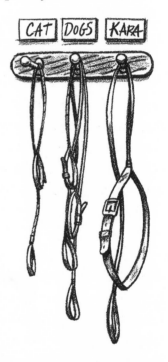

The hardest part about all these therapies was the illusion I clung to that they could somehow repair the damage. I was acutely annoyed that they were attempting to teach me how to do things differently instead of just getting me back to how I did them before. It was a long time before I realized that the application of successful compensatory techniques and healing were almost the same.

April was important because I finally found the rage everyone had been displaying on my behalf. From the onset, I was not angry with the woman who had hit me. I assumed she felt bad and I kept thinking how I would have felt if I had been responsible for an accident like ours. When I saw her in the hospital, she was almost hysterical. She was apologizing and sobbing and I really felt for her.

Until April 9TH.

I was subpoenaed to testify at her ticket hearing. It was the first time I had worn a suit since the accident and I realized how much weight I was gaining. I also remembered how much I hated wearing nylons.

I was pretty nervous. I had never been in a courtroom before and the shiny walls of heavy wood intimidated me. A dozen or so people were called before me and many of them could not speak English. They were answering to charges involving drunk and reckless driving, entering the freeway via the exit ramp and exceeding the speed limit by more than 20 MPH. They asked for fewer points, more lenient fines and reduced probation, mostly through interpreters. When the judge didn't appear to be alarmed that these people could not read road signs written in English, and when he casually granted their requests one after another, Diana and I couldn't believe it.

The woman who hit me pleaded "guilty with an explanation." She told the judge that even though she ran *two* red lights, it was *my fault* (pause for effect) because ... *I should have seen her.* She said that had I been paying attention, this would never have happened. She also said that she had seen me in the hospital and that I was "fine." Presumably her idea of "fine" is an ambulance escort on a backboard with a cervical collar and blipping machines and scurrying doctors. Go figure.

Even though the officer spoke on my behalf and produced witness testimony supporting her liability for my injuries, she was fined merely $125 for court costs. Her record would be cleared of this "incident" if she could remain accident-free for the next two years. She asked for a lighter sentence (imagine!), but was denied due to her *number of prior accidents*.

She did not understand the first thing about a head injury. She didn't realize that it was her choice to end the life I'd had, not mine. She didn't know how it felt to wake up every morning with a headache. Or what it's like to not have any balance. Or what it feels like to lose a career, an independent lifestyle, and the ability to drive. She wasn't sitting at home wondering how long it would be before they foreclosed on her home. She wasn't living her life on Post-it notes. She could drive and she could work and she could put this all behind her.

Her sentence would last two years. Mine would last a lifetime.

I'll Carry the Fork!

LEARNING TO SUCCEED

June 4, 1996

I was standing in line at Target. All of a sudden, I was furious with the young woman behind the register. I just wanted to KILL her! I don't know why. Diana ended up taking me home. I'm so embarrassed.

June 10, 1996

So today was Dr. Cini, and I must say she shoots straight from the hip. Honest, powerfully honest. Yet calm and comforting and patient. She talked about medical disability for life, perhaps. She talked about acceptance and reality and considering options. I didn't have time to let it all sink in. I was off then, putting on smiles and reporting the news to my friends like an objective observer. Not feeling, not allowing, not absorbing. But it is patient and it waits and it doesn't change. And then Wham! It hits you and there are tears and you wonder: what the hell am I going to do? I keep trying to be up and to laugh and to be strong and it just seems like the farther I get down the road, the darker and colder and scarier it becomes. And I think, OK, soon it'll start rolling my way. But the time between even minuscule points of progress lasts seemingly for years and slowly I move farther away from the life I had and, without even realizing it, closer to a new one I am already creating. I am crying now and I don't care and it seems like I'm just not going to stop.

It's a real curse, this "mild head injury." You are just well enough to realize what isn't well. The better you feel, the more you do; the more you do, the more you realize what you cannot do any longer. Subtle things. Things that only you notice. Or maybe other people do, and they just don't have the heart to point them out.

And others didn't understand. How could they? They couldn't see the hundred and one things I was doing behind the scenes to present myself as normal. I looked the same (except for the extra poundage). I didn't talk on the phone or entertain guests when my speech was really bad or my head was breaking concrete. I nodded through conversations. I was scared to admit to myself, much less to them, that things were really wrong. I still felt that "mild" meant minor and that I was a failure, somehow, for not being better by then.

How could I expect them to understand when I hadn't? As kids, we were always catching line drives with our foreheads and falling off our bikes trying to pop wheelies. Our parents were told to wake us up every hour and ask us how many fingers they were holding up. That was the extent of head injury as we knew it.

And yet it continued. I would watch rain come pouring through my open window without any inclination to shut it. If somebody didn't call or visit, it was as if they did not exist. Even my family. I'd walk into a room and have no idea what I had just intended to do. I would listen to my television and realize how low the volume was but wouldn't think to turn it up.

I had horrible flashbacks. I'd close my eyes and hear the blunt impact. The dull twisting of metal and plastic. The sudden silence. I could smell the oxygen mask. I could hear the sound of my jeans ripping as they were cut off me. I could feel the somber eyes of people at the scene watching me being pulled from my car and strapped to a board.

I got angry at nothing. One night something irked me and I tore down the wallpaper in my living room. I interrupted people. They could tell me that they had just found the cure for cancer and I would cut them off and talk about how pretty the car next to us was.

As for riding in cars ... my poor friends! Going through intersections was a white-knuckle event, probably more so for the driver than for me. I would be slamming my "brake" on the floor of the passenger's side or digging my nails into their upholstery. I told one of my drivers once that if he was going to continue to press the gas pedal while I was "braking," we were going to drop the transmission!

At times I imagined my mind a devilish child. CDs and books that I did not recall ordering would arrive in the mail. Pizzas would show up unannounced, or the pizza place would call and ask if I *reeeeeally* wanted both the identical pizzas I had ordered 10 minutes apart.

I was getting better at finding ways to approach these problems, though. After killing all my houseplants, I started marking every Wednesday on my calendar as Plant Watering Day. I designated one light in my house to signal that I was doing laundry. Instead of finding damp, musty clothes in the washer three days later, I knew if that particular light was on to check the machine.

I still found sandwiches in the cupboard and salad bowls in the linen closet. My friend Kris cautiously asked if I knew there were kitchen utensils in my freezer. I still poured cream in my water at restaurants. I still fell when I didn't concentrate on my balance. And I still walked right out in front of cars when I *did*.

I was scaring people, I knew. But I was determined not to have someone come and live with me. I knew if I was going to hang on to my last bit of independence, I would have to distinguish between pride and stupidity. Between struggling to do what I could and conceding what I knew I couldn't. I would need to eliminate the things I was doing that were dangerous. Like falling out of my shower when I tilted my head back to rinse my hair ... falling off a chair and landing on the stove just trying to change a light bulb ... breaking my hand when I fell one day while dusting. (My friends saw an opportunity here: they told their husbands that dusting was just too dangerous and they shouldn't take the chance of hurting themselves.)

I had a devil of a time trying to remember when I had something in the oven. I would cook and cook and cook until the fire alarm would tell me it was done. If it hadn't been for my friends, I would have starved, burned my house down, or acquired "canned-potato disorder."

I finally decided to heed my therapists' advice and equip my shower with a seat, a guardrail and a hand nozzle. I decided I wouldn't change light bulbs or clean my ceiling fans. I stopped crossing busy streets during rush hour and I grudgingly (ha!) gave up dusting. I knew I couldn't sit all day in front of the oven just to make sure I didn't forget I was cooking. So I decided, *I'll carry the fork!* to remind me. I think I heard a collective sigh of relief from everyone who had worried for my safety. In fact, I felt a little relieved myself: I was finding ways, even if they were occasionally a little bizarre, to start to cope.

The Red Wings,
Billy Joel and
the Symphony Orchestra

LIFE ON THE ISLAND

May 30, 1996

To hell with 'em! ... I'll cure myself then.

It bothered me that I still couldn't sing. I was embarrassed by how I stuck on words and stuttered through them. My friends were great; they never made me feel self-conscious. They laughed, yes. But just to let me know everything was going to work out, whether I healed entirely or not. They would guess the words sometimes. Or I would describe what I was trying to say and they would figure it out. When I got nervous or tired or excited, my words would rush and bump into each other like bargain-hunting shoppers on the day after Christmas.

I picked one of the hardest songs I know, "Scenes from an Italian Restaurant," by Billy Joel. The song is fast, the tempo changes and it is difficult to get all the words out clearly, even for someone without a speech impediment. I was determined this would fix me so I started playing that song 15, 20 times a night. Lord only knows what the neighbors thought. I would sing it over and over and over. I was horrible. Frustrated. During one of my more "inappropriate" moments, I tore the doors and the back off my entertainment center. Pretty.

But I was nothing if not persistent. I kept playing that song, convinced I was going to make progress. Slowly, the words came. I kept up with them longer and more consistently. I was able to change speed, anticipate the tempo, and 32 days later (I counted), I sang, "Scenes from an Italian Restaurant" for the first time from start to finish without a mistake. I broke down and cried.

Thinking I was cured for sure, I wrote a letter to Billy Joel, thanking him for his silent part in my recovery. A week later it was returned; I had sent it to the wrong address. Good thing, because I had sealed the envelope *minus the letter*. So much for the great recovery.

I've often thought that if you're going to sustain an injury that will take away your ability to drive, it's best to do it in a town with a great sports team. (Bet you thought I was going to say public transportation system!) I promised myself that I would not get hooked on soap operas, although my friends were incredulous that I would pass up such an opportunity. Instead, I tuned in to Rosie or Oprah and I watched every hockey game the Detroit Red Wings played. Because I spent so much time in my house and on my own, I would have gone crazy without them.

It was difficult, though. In addition to my inappropriate anger, I also wept uncontrollably. Watching the Red Wings in the Stanley Cup playoffs was an emotional roller coaster. I would cry through the national anthem. I would cry every time we scored and any time the crowd cheered. Almost wracking sobs, mind you. A minute later I would be cursing and throwing the remote because the other team scored or the ref missed a call. I stopped watching games with my friends because I was such a lunatic. Thank goodness the Wings won a record 62 games that season. I was running out of furniture.

When I wasn't singing or watching the Red Wings, I was trying just about everything to reconnect the damaged pathways crisscrossing my brain. Aunt Fredda had heard that playing the keyboard was a great exercise for coordinating brain functions, so I started sounding out songs. Because it was hockey season, I learned "O, Canada" and played it on my friends' answering machines. I colored and painted by numbers.

I tried to stimulate feeling in my feet by walking in rice and sawdust. Every morning I would run warm and cold water on them. I did my stretches and my therapy homework. When I hit a problem, I tried to invent a solution. If that didn't work, I tried to reduce the anger and frustration by just eliminating the offending activity from my life. Probably a good thing I wasn't having trouble breathing.

People were great. My cousins, Kris and Linda, drove more than eight hours just to check on me, offer therapeutic massage and suggest the benefits of acupuncture. Cherie became a Reiki master and attempted to help me with ancient rituals. Christine sent sage and cedar from Denver to cleanse and purify me. Aunt Phyllis brought me magnetic pillows and blankets and mattress pads to sleep with. A woman I'd just met in a coffeehouse offered me the business card of a homeopathic healer who worked with herbal combinations. Whatever cures people had heard of, they told me and I tried them—except for the cabdriver, bless his heart, who told me that ballet lessons would cure my balance problem. Even a head injury was not going to get me into a tutu.

Although I talk about attorneys and their significance in a later chapter, one of the most important things my attorney ever did for me had nothing to do with litigation.

Six months into my recovery, I was still bewildered by the idea that this was a "mild" injury and that tests indicated no serious damage. Though several doctors subsequently criticized that diagnosis, given to me by one of the specialists I saw for a few minutes early on, the term stuck. We live in a society that registers blood and stitches and bruises and crutches as proof of injury and I was no different. In the absence of those obvious props, I started to wonder if I was going crazy. You think, My God! It's not *bad enough?* There's not *enough damage?* That's like telling a family that just lost their home to an earthquake that it's no big deal, the quake didn't register very high on the Richter scale.

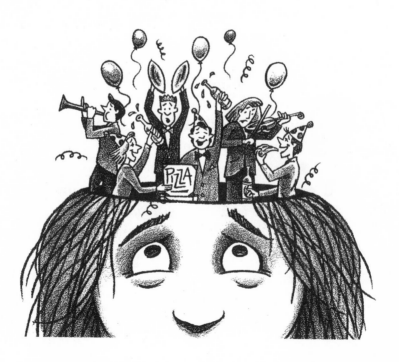

My attorney wrote me a letter and likened my injury to a symphony orchestra. He said the tests could tell you if all the trumpet players were present or if the string section was accounted for, but they could not tell you how well the musicians communicated with the conductor, or how each individual was playing. He explained that with a head injury, all the musicians might be present, but some might not be playing, or not in the right key. Finally, I was starting to understand. I imagined that half my orchestra was playing Beethoven and the rest of those lazy bastards were in the dressing room eating pizza.

My speech therapist told me that the term "mild" described the severity of the injury, not the duration of recovery. That was important. She told me that I could experience "mild" symptoms for years, maybe permanently. A lot would heal, most likely, as my brain recovered and the nerves and connectors found new pathways to determine and detect messages. But she cautioned there was no way of telling just how long it would take or how much would return.

One of my doctors explained that if my brain were a house (mine was most likely a *messy* house), everything I knew before the accident was in storage down hallways and behind closed doors. The theory was that even though an earthquake might rock the foundation, I still had that information. I just needed to go down those hallways, pry open the doors, turn on the lights and sift through those rooms. It would take time.

I cannot say enough about those doctors and therapists and attorneys who kept searching for stories and other ways to describe the effects of brain trauma. They were like teachers with a troubled student, trying to find new ways to say the same thing. They suspected, as I did, that understanding as much as I could about the injury would help my acceptance of, compensation for and recovery from it. When you're catapulted into your first significant injury, you're instantly behind the eight ball in more ways than one. It's like lacing up skates for the first time—then going out to play goalie in the Stanley Cup finals.

Of course, those goalies are said to be a little off the wall anyway. Maybe we're onto something here.

Loving All My PETS
But This One

UNDERSTANDING "PAIN AND SUFFERING"

July 23, 1996

The young man and I chatted easily about the beautiful Upper Peninsula. He was originally from Louisville and was planning to backpack up near Pictured Rocks.

I eagerly stoked the conversation with questions about his decision to attend school and we talked about the respected reputation of Wayne State University. As I chatted along, I made myself oblivious to the needle biting my arm as the young man displayed the skills of his internship.

They laid a heated sheet of pliable plastic over my face, with holes arranged around my eyes, nose and mouth. As it cooled, it formed a firm mask they could fasten to the table by the edges so that I wouldn't move. Soothingly, they told me that I would need to remain still during the test, as they secured my arms with tightened straps across my ribs, eliminating any other possibility of movement.

The "pictures" would take 20 minutes, during which time I could not move. The first 10 minutes or so were easy. I imagined I resembled Hannibal Lector in *Silence of the Lambs*.

But slowly, gradually, the back of my head became numb and my fingers and feet tingled. I lay on what felt like a great mass, unable to distinguish between my head and neck. My nose itched and I told myself (mind over matter!) it would go away.

The pressure on the lower back of my head became almost intolerable. I told myself they would come soon, and I strained to see them behind the safety glass that protected them from radioactivity.

When they finally came and removed the mask, my head was numb and I shook my hands to chase away the pins and needles.

They changed the IV and put a pillow behind my head, dimming the lights as they left the room. Here I would stay, quiet and still for 30 minutes, while my body absorbed the dripping stranger.

My mind dozed. I wondered how my brain looked in neon. I glanced at the clock. It had now been an hour and a half since this whole ordeal started.

When they returned, the pillow was removed and the mask and straps returned. I felt like I had been paroled, and now my return to solitary was frightening because this time I knew what the next 20 minutes would entail.

The pressure increased quickly this time, my hands and feet tingling almost immediately. There was no relief; I could not move. My eyes watered. I blinked away the tears so I could see the clock on the right wall. I mentally counted the minutes.

I was sweating now. I began to panic. I struggled to raise my head, even just a fraction, to relieve the pressure. I could not.

I fought the panic. I pictured being anywhere but there. I closed my eyes. I told myself that it would be over. That I could do it.

My mouth started to water and I thought I would vomit. I looked to the window and one of the women was talking on the phone. She was keeping tabs on me, and I mentally counted the time it would take for her to realize I was in trouble if I threw up while lying on my back beneath a mask with my arms bound.

I knew then why they call the night before a PET scan for "next of kin" emergency numbers. I also knew why, unlike the MRI and CT scans, they bound your arms and did not give you an emergency button. I would have been all over that table like a fish on land, pushing the button till all of Nuclear Medicine knew this hurt like hell. It was like having the back of your head slowly impaled. The term "pain and suffering" lawyers use when seeking damages in injury cases took on vivid new meaning.

I also understood why they don't tell you quite everything, because after that first time I would have been out the door, down the hall and halfway home before they came at me with that mask.

I fought not to call out and tell them to stop the test. I told myself that if the test was invalidated, I would forfeit the chance they would find something in me to fix. And I knew I would not agree to another test, couldn't go through this again, if this first test was compromised.

When they finally came in and removed the mask and the straps, I wiped the sweat from my face. I felt my jeans cling to the back of my legs and my shirt was damp. I sat up, regaining my balance and tapping my feet together to restore the feeling.

We exchanged pleasantries as they walked me to the door and wished me well. I went outside, found a grassy hill, sat down and cried.

Confidence, Esteem
and Consciousness

BE TRUE TO YOUR SELVES

August 4, 1996

It was late July. The summer had been mild, so this afternoon of mid-90 degree temperatures and wilting humidity really took my breath away. I was walking home, laboring from the heat and suffering from an ego that would not let me call someone to pick me up.

As I approached a Dairy Queen, I saw a little girl holding a woman's hand. The resemblance was unmistakable: mother and daughter. The little girl turned my way, her eyes magnetically pulled to my cane.

Her eyes were big with wonder and curiosity. Eyes that asked, "Mommy, what's that?" Eyes that did not yet judge, not yet criticize, not yet ridicule.

I smiled. A warm, welcoming smile. If I had been in line behind them, perhaps I might have bent down and said hello. I might have let her hold my cane, twirling it like a baton, giggling away the stigma. I would have delighted in the innocence that knows no prejudice.

In front of her face appeared a tiny cone of swirled chocolate that soon would run down the sides before she could catch it with her tongue. Her mother, looking down to see why her daughter had not taken the cone from her, followed the line of her beautiful eyes until she saw me, inching along in the afternoon sun.

She took her child's head between thumb and fingers and sharply snapped it toward the wall. She bent down, and in a voice meant perhaps to apologize to me, said, "You don't stare at cripples!"

The good thing about being disabled (or, as I prefer, "differently abled") is that you never have to worry about your appearance. You can stop wearing makeup. Stop shaving your legs. Let your eyebrows connect in the middle. You don't have to brush your hair, or even wash it. You can wear bunny slippers to restaurants, match stripes with plaids, or go naked as the day you were born. Because the second you sit in a wheelchair or use a walker or take up a cane or attach braces to limbs or patches to eyes, everyone stops looking at you.

I imagine that little girl with the ice cream cone will grow up automatically diverting her eyes to the floor in the presence of disability. She will be taught that people with physical and cognitive impairments are to be looked away from, stepped aside for, treated as invisible or, if unavoidably noticed, viewed with beagle-eyed pity.

When I was walking home one day, two teenagers on bikes rode by and yelled, "Fucking re-*tarrrd!*" One well-meaning man told me I should get a three-wheeler so I wouldn't have to walk everywhere. Then he paused and said, "But no, then people would think you're retarded." How nice.

Our self-worth and self-esteem are tied so terribly tightly to our careers and possessions and physical appearance, and by how we measure up to the people next door, at the next desk or next in line. We hide behind suits and titles and gauge our importance by how high up the ladder we've ascended. We tally points for how many *things* we've accumulated, how expensive a car we drive, how big a house we own. We are judged by our manicured lawns and our platinum lines of credit. By the standard of youth and beauty. By our ability to eliminate or hide the effects of age. We are a society that binds, colors, tucks, hides and trims everything about us that makes us who we are, everything that reflects the entirety of our experiences. We worship the kind of beauty that comes from bottles, creams, pills and lotions. And we discard those who become too old, too weak, too damaged, too fat, too ugly or too poor.

I was a successful catering manager before my accident. Losing my job and my career was a blow I was ill-prepared to handle. Accepting that I would probably never play basketball or dance freely again made me confront a reality that arrived 50 years too soon. Half a century before I expected it. The idea that I might never drive again, at the age of 32, was incomprehensible. Utilizing a cane to ambulate safely, and equipping my home and lifestyle to accommodate the changes in my health and abilities, were unwelcome reminders that sometimes the future comes right up your steps, pounds on the door, and forces its way in whether you're dressed and ready to meet it or not.

I gained 30 pounds before I stopped counting. While doctors worried about dizziness when I bent to tie my shoes, I worried that I would asphyxiate myself. I had these disgusting growths on my face from the medication I was taking. My breasts were lactating at one point. I was stooped over and shuffling around with the cane. If you get the feeling I was having a hard time finding the inspiration to get out of the house and participate in the new life assigned to me— you're right.

The recovery process is a fine example of the "long and winding road" made famous by the Beatles' song. At the beginning, we're so adamant about returning quickly to the life we had. It's hurry, hurry, hurry and fix me so I can get back to everything I've created and everything I've known. The system immediately sweeps you up, informing you of an injury you don't understand and refuse to believe. It convinces you until you finally trade denial for acceptance. Then it sends you to more professionals to make sure you're not lying. To keep your expectations realistic, the system is very guarded in its optimism and attempts to keep your optimism in check, too. A few months down the road, it sends you to more professionals to find out why you feel so hopeless and depressed.

The process starts with a shining mountain called "expectation of recovery," slides down into a valley where no hope blossoms, and eventually evens out somewhere on the side of the road when you get off the bus and make your own decision about where you really want to travel. You have to get past the point of realizing you can't go back but not yet knowing how to go forward. In the privacy of your own thoughts you find yourself battling naked, stripped of the armor you once hid behind, left to survive on the rations of a self-identity that feels as bare as Mother Hubbard's cupboard.

Advice for climbing the mountain called success is abundantly available. There's no shortage of experts to tell us what clothes to wear and what stocks to purchase and what courses to take and what foods to eat. Apply this moisturizer. Try these running shoes. Take these vitamins. Save this amount for retirement by the time you're 30.

But we don't offer fluffy pillows for soft landings when people stumble off that mountain. The rate of suicide and violence and depression in this country is astounding for those who don't make the grade. Oh, you're a model who just turned 40? Sorry. Hey you, over there, the pitcher who's lost the heat on his fastball: see ya! Oh, wow, sorry you were downsized by a computer seven months before retirement. Lost your legs while serving our country overseas? Tough break, man! For these we have no vitamins or moisturizers or easy answers.

One of the most important steps in recovering from any traumatic event is realizing you need help—that you can't always make it by yourself—and finding the strength to seek it out. Somewhere along the way, pride becomes not only stifling but also dangerous. A blow to the head means a blow to the ego, self-esteem and confidence of the victim. And these symptoms, unlike those of memory and attention, are likely to become worse when left untreated.

It only took seconds to sustain a head injury. But it took days to name it, weeks to deny it and months to understand it. My independence was gone. Not only did I depend on my parents for money and my friends for food and transportation, I had to realize and accept the importance of people who specialize in brain injury. I had to put my bull-headedness aside long enough to allow the doctors and attorneys and therapists to help me put my life back together.

We've got to stop snapping our children's heads to the wall in the face of disability. If we teach them that "different" cannot even be acknowledged, much less welcomed, what will we be able to tell them if they're unfortunate enough to end up on the bus?

Too many people become senselessly damaged and cognitively disabled by head injury. We cannot afford to let young minds be senselessly damaged by misguided fear and prejudice.

Double Take

GRIEVING THE LOSS

My Therapist

She is my full-length mirror
With a voice.
My honest mechanic,
Fixing even those things I don't know to be wrong.
She is a mile-marker in my marathon,
My safari guide to uncharted feelings,
The interpreter in the language of my life.
My therapist is the one in my corner who believes enough
To never step in and stop the fight.
She is my rear view mirror,
Warning that objects in my past may be closer
Than they appear.
My therapist is my calendar,
Reminding me that spring follows winter.
She is my interior decorator,
Helping to polish the structure I have built.

Therapists. Once considered mainly the paid companions of the wealthy, they have crossed the bridge from trendy luxury to household necessity. The microwaves of the '90s: accessible means of bringing quick warmth to shivering souls.

My friend Christine, a therapist in Denver, called to tell me that she had heard a psychologist speak on the importance of psychotherapy in recovering from brain injury. Although I was willing to sing praises about therapy as a tool in understanding one's past and dissecting patterns of behavior in relationships, I was not quite certain how my therapist was going to help me overcome the physical, behavioral and cognitive challenges I now faced.

I knew brain injuries to be as distinct and discrete as the people who sustained them. I suspected that effective treatment and support, though probably outlined in some "how to" manual for mental health professionals, would demand an open mind from both of us.

I was fortunate to have a therapist who not only anticipated my success, but was also extremely patient and good-humored. She would be tested.

The problems associated with brain injury are complex and far-reaching. They run the gamut from acceptance to adjustment to depression to loss of identity and self-esteem, and the priorities—figuring out where to start—can be as incoherent as the injured brain itself. I had my therapist, Ginger Keena, metaphorically juggling bowling balls and flaming torches, and her challenge was not to drop any regardless of the distractions I provided.

I considered our sessions to be escapes from the medical battle I was waging, reprieves from the stoic soldier I had become. I had (prematurely) buried the feelings of self-pity and grief in the company of those who continued to remind me how "lucky" I was. Ginger encouraged me to allow those feelings to surface and to examine them without fear of guilt or repercussion. Gradually we began to integrate the compartments labeled "my injury" and "my life." It wasn't easy.

When I vacillated between the extremes of either minimizing my injury or being consumed by it, she urged me to lay it right out on the table and really *look* at it. By acknowledging its impact on my life, and by having a safe and consistent environment to work in, I was able to start getting some perspective of life beyond the injury. But it was a long process.

I have to give Ginger much of the credit. Before the accident, I would often come into therapy with notes or well-thought-out ideas on a topic or two I wanted to discuss. I would devote serious thought to this, determining in detail the avenue we would pursue during our session. Our conversations were intelligent. (Well, her side of our conversations was intelligent.) We had some measure of focus. We could track where we had come from and, often, where we were heading. It felt sane, progressive and logical.

After the accident, I was not the same client. Our sessions were no longer chess matches of like thinkers contemplating and discussing important moves and decisions in my life. They were now more like Chinese fire drills. New Year's Eve at Times Square. Painted, plastic horses on merry-go-rounds. Ginger, I imagine, was just plain bewildered; I know I was. More than once she wrapped up our time with, "Well, we were certainly all over the place today." Diplomatically put.

My lists now came on neon paper with pretty pictures. I wanted to cover 20 different topics in one hour. While she was concerned about how I was handling the prospect of using a wheelchair, I found myself concerned that her switch plates didn't match, or a picture was tilted, or the chairs were not right. In the middle of a discussion on self-doubt or my feelings of incompetence, I would interrupt her and go off on a totally different tangent. I would talk, talk, talk about something and then lose the entire idea. Sometimes she would stop me and say, "Kara, I'm not really following you." Other times I would stop in midsentence and ask, "What the hell am I talking about?"

We had a lot of ground to cover. I had been a preaccident workaholic, so special attention was paid to the effect of this extended period without working. Whatever you're inclined to believe, an extended medical leave is not enviable. It's no vacation in the Bahamas. The importance of having a job and going to work and earning a paycheck is significant. The satisfaction that comes from success in work is horribly conspicuous in its absence. After an injury that requires extensive care, a sense of purpose and focus often gives way to a listless lack of direction. You lose not only your ability to work, but also the mentality and conditioning of a worker.

It wasn't until after my accident that I understood how so many retired people could be busy all the time, yet never seem to get much accomplished. People spend 30, 40 years getting up at the crack of dawn, working all day, going to their kids' ball games, bowling on Thursdays. Then they retire, and suddenly reading the newspaper can take all morning. You lose your routines and rituals, timetables and deadlines. One day you realize that having your clothes pressed and your hair done have lost their importance. You find little in common with people who are at work, dreading work, or talking about work. I observed that I had become quite content in my flannels, telling friends what my dogs had done that day.

Another source of frustration was that neither Ginger nor I knew which symptoms or problems were the result of my injury, and which were actually the result of the recovery process. It sometimes felt like splitting hairs to try and distinguish which causes were responsible for which effect. Neither of us knew enough about brain injury to decipher its subtleties. But Ginger had known me before my accident, and more than anyone else was able to compare the person I was becoming to the person I had been.

I was embarrassed any time one of my doctors asked what my daily routine entailed. I would get up and read the paper with a ruler, going from line to line. Then I'd wait however long it took for the mail to come. I might take a shower and walk to the 7-11 to get toilet paper and a can of soup. Since I had trouble remembering a story line for long, I would find a movie that I had already seen and watch it the four or five times it was on cable that month. My dad would call and ask what day it was. Or I would. My afternoon nap would get me ready for the Wings' game and then *wowee!* Another day gone. At three or four in the morning, I would be ready to take on the world.

I was, for all intents and purposes, retired at the age of 32. At times I even recognized that I was not heading entirely in the right direction.

Unattractive realities reared their ugly little heads. Accepting the fact that I was needy and dependent on others, when I had prided myself on independence and self-sufficiency, was one of the most difficult challenges. Learning to ask for help and allow myself to be helped were lessons I would have preferred to learn in smaller doses. They represent battles that, quite frankly, I will never claim to have fully won.

I traded safety for stupidity more times than I'll admit. I was stubborn beyond reason and damned lucky I never injured myself more seriously than I did. Sometimes I would lie to my friends and tell them so-and-so was coming over to take me grocery shopping. Then I would spend the next six hours walking a mile to the store, shopping for more things than I could possibly carry, resting under some tree or by the side of a road, and walking back home. Did I mention the 90 degree weather?

I just wanted to prove I could *do* things. Things that would challenge even "normal" people.

I conjured up creative ways to avoid asking for help. I found a place that delivered groceries to your home if you ordered food from their restaurant. So some days during the win- 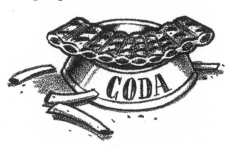 ter when I couldn't walk, I ordered rib dinners and hamburgers just to get cream for my coffee. I didn't even *like* their ribs. The dogs ate well.

I ordered everything from Christmas presents to shampoo out of catalogs. People would call and thank me for the brownies and cheese boards UPS had delivered, and I would secretly hope that what I sent them was what I intended. That first Christmas I was so discombobulated with whom I'd sent what that I rang up quite a hefty sum. I am proud to report that I am now on the Swiss Colony Elite-Client Tasting Board of Governors—admittedly not an ambition I had ever consciously harbored, but hey! How many can make *that* claim?

I suppose it was half ego and half denial that kept me from accepting that I could no longer take care of everything myself. You have no idea how many trips you take to the corner for milk or eggs or coffee or cat litter—until you can't. I needed so *much* help—especially during those first six months—and I resented it. Waiting for people to come and enable me to do things I had done all my life was horribly frustrating. I had to jump from one extreme to another: exceptional (maybe even ornery) independence to exceptional (and definitely ornery) dependence. Admittedly, I could have—perhaps should have—allowed people to participate more in my life before the accident. After the accident, they weren't merely participating; they were living it, keeping it warm and pounding its chest until I came back to reclaim it.

I found myself further frustrated with the fact that the doctors and specialists were treating little parts of me and only Dr. Cini, my primary care physician, was trying to keep all the pieces together. Doctor A would see me once and then six months later. Specialist B would schedule me for a test and I'd never see him again. I felt like a car at the Ford assembly plant. Everyone does his or her little part, but no one sees the whole. Just tighten her screws and roll her down the line.

Thankfully, I was treated by only one psychotherapist. That helped. Constant assessment of my abilities in physical therapy had allowed me to ascertain my progress in mobility and strength. Psychotherapy provided a comparable measure of my emotional status, a way to recognize and build on mental progress.

Psychotherapy also covered areas that traditional medical treatment could not. When Dr. Cini ordered a PET scan to determine possible causes of inappropriate anger in the frontal lobe of the brain, Ginger worked with me to identify any emotional triggers for such behavior. It was like tag-team treatment. I felt that nothing was being left uncovered.

Sometimes I wondered how I would ever get my "worker mindset" back. I often wondered how I ever worked at all.

Where I was first so impatient about how long everything was taking, I eventually surrendered to it. I was waiting for something to end this period in my life. Frequently I found myself lying on my couch, just waiting: waiting for my old life to come back and reclaim me.

Ginger was always supportive of positive thinking and hope, but she guided me down the difficult road of honesty and reality that well-meaning friends and family members didn't have the heart to follow. She asked tough questions. She explored the less favorable scenarios, the ones I didn't care to hear, the ones I couldn't *imagine* accepting—like the one that said some of my injuries might be permanent.

The benefits of integrating psychotherapy into overall recovery cannot be overstated. It may be group support, individual counseling, or a combination of both. Because I had spent a great deal of time feeling guilty for my grief, and selfish for appearing ungrateful when I was so "lucky," I thought group therapy would be less helpful for me. I knew I would probably be surrounded by people who were more severely injured than I had been, and I imagined I would bury my real feelings out of respect for their more difficult challenges. Sure, I might stop feeling sorry for myself, but I also knew that individual therapy was providing me the only real outlet for the sadness and anger I needed to purge. And there were extra helpings of both.

I hated my inability to drive. I hated the fact that I could no longer play basketball. I hated the pictures on my wall that taunted me with the person I had been. People would joke that I should install a towrope to the corner, or hitch up the dogs and sled to the store when it snowed. I laughed; I knew they were only trying to keep me laughing. But it stung. The kind of hurt that burns the cheeks and quivers the lip. The kind of hurt that waits until everyone is gone, and you're alone and fragile, to pounce on you with foot-long claws.

There were times I just wanted to lash out at someone! When I kept telling my physical therapist that I planned on playing ball again, she suggested I stand with my back to a wall and dribble. Or stand in my hallway and throw the ball against the opposite wall, playing catch with myself. "How utterly ridiculous," I thought.

She also suggested, as Ginger and so many others did, that I try wheelchair basketball. They were trying to ignite the athletic competitiveness I had always displayed. But I wasn't ready to go there. Sometimes it was all I could do to not tell them all to go to hell!

The movie *Brian's Song* is about a young Chicago Bears' football player battling cancer. It's one of my all-time favorites. There's a scene where the doctor is telling Brian Piccolo they have found more of the tumor and they have to operate again. Brian becomes angry and refuses to sign the papers authorizing surgery. Gale Sayers pulls the doctor aside and explains to him how a ballplayer prepares both physically and mentally for a game; how he has his own inner timetable so that, when the game starts, he is at peak performance level. He explains to the doctor that Brian just isn't ready yet, that he needs a little more time to prepare.

I kept hearing things I wasn't ready to hear yet, and I needed a little more time to prepare.

Brain injury support counseling doesn't just help accident survivors. It is invaluable to families and friends who find it difficult to understand how the lives and relationships of their loved ones have changed. It's also an opportunity for survivors to share insights about compensatory techniques that might help in daily activities. (That's how I learned about the timer for taking my "candy.") It's a chance to find helpful associations, attorneys who specialize in head trauma, and reading materials that shed light on how the process unfolds. It affords survivors and their families an opportunity to meet other people who got on the bus before them, and who might know the shortcuts and detours down the road.

Although I enthusiastically support some form of professional counseling for survivors, I am not convinced that a therapist must specialize in head trauma to be helpful. Early on, one specialist seemed to scoff at my level of damage (at least that's the impression I got). I could see her from the waiting room. She was wearing some God-awful, brownish suit and barking orders at her assistant. I called her the "Butterscotch Bitch." After she graciously spent all of seven minutes with me, she waved her hand, almost discarding me, and told me I had "nothing to worry about." I asked her what my X-rays revealed and she said, "Oh, a spot and a space, nothing to concern yourself over." When I could not recall the word "umbrella," which she had told me to remember as a test, she said, "It's the thing you take with you to shield you from the rain." Then I said "umbrella," and she said, "Good, your short-term memory is unaffected." Huh?

She spoke of the countless others she had treated, giving me the impression my injury paled by comparison. At that point, all I knew was that I only had one brain and it had been injured. Whether damage was or wasn't serious in her eyes didn't matter to me. It was my damage, it would change my life and I resented the implication that *that* wasn't serious.

Ginger was not trained specifically to counsel head injury survivors. In some ways, that was good. She didn't know any more than I did about brain trauma, but she knew *me.* In a sense she had fewer weapons to bring to the battle than a specialist, but more ammunition. As I pulled myself through the knothole of brain injury, she was able to help me recognize which parts made it through unscathed, which were a little battered and which didn't make it at all.

She was not inclined to compare me to other people with brain injuries, so neither was I. She was willing to learn about the injury from me and for me, so symptoms weren't assumed or suggested. We could deal with the actual facts of my situation. She provided a much-needed space separate from the hospitals and rehab centers that consumed my new life. And the vision that some semblance of normalcy waited for me beyond this current existence made my sessions with her feel like R&R ports to a battle-weary ship.

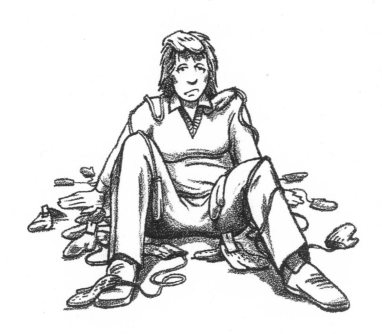

My falls were terribly embarrassing. The first time I cabbed to the mall by myself, I misjudged the moving step on the escalator and tumbled straight down to the lower level. I took out a mitten display at K-Mart; the lawn equipment wall at the hardware store; the louvered door that left me lying in my heater room. Diana would unlock my side of the car and by the time she got to the driver's side I was nowhere to be found. Just like that.

I didn't want to fall in front of Ginger. I don't know why that was so important. Maybe because I had fallen in front of just about everyone else. Maybe because she anticipated my success so staunchly and I wanted to nurture that belief. I wanted to step inside her office and leave the injury outside the door. Whatever the reason, I was especially careful in her presence.

Then, when I was leaving one day, I paused to adjust my backpack before going outside. Here comes Ginger, right through the door, and there goes Kara. Her shock (fear?) and my embarrassment must have kept us both from laughing or crying. Here's the one person I wanted least to fall in front of, and I stand right in front of an exit door adjusting my backpack. Good thinking.

There are two frontiers to recovery from any traumatic injury. The emotional damage must be dealt with as diligently as the physical damage. Each area has the ability to strengthen or weaken the other.

Medical professionals can't and won't guarantee complete recovery, and in the interests of conservatism, may project unduly dismal scenarios. Families and friends can't bring themselves to accept anything less than complete recovery, and in the interests of protecting everyone's emotions, may project unduly rosy scenarios. Psychotherapy looks for the solid ground between these two extremes. It acknowledges best- and worst-case scenarios, but reduces fear by helping the patient understand that reality will most likely fall somewhere between the two.

While medical doctors were helping me recover my lost physical balance, Ginger was helping me recover perspective, self-esteem and direction: my emotional balance.

188 Days Till Payday

POWER OF ATTORNEY

March 12, 1996

I will never need money to pay for my funeral ... they've already buried me in paperwork.

Diana and Marty brought food and bones for the dogs. Diana spent her whole day off cooking me enough food for two weeks of meals. I am running out of thank-yous. They are spending all this money on me and it just isn't right.

September 16, 1996

Debora took me downtown so I would be closer to a cab. Cabbed to Ginger's. Little Dianna picked me up and brought me back to the DIA [Detroit Institute of Arts]. Waited till Bill got off work and he came and brought me home. I can't afford to cab everywhere. I don't know what else to do.

In the week following my accident, I received flowers and cards and visits from family, friends and people I worked with. They sent surprise packages, food and called all the time to check up on me. It was a wonderful outpouring of genuine warmth.

Their lavish support was a bit unexpected. But the amount of attention I received from attorneys wishing to handle my case was downright astonishing. Given that my case made no headlines and did not rock the world (other than mine), their ability to find me seemed most curious. After half a dozen letters with calling cards arrived in the mail that first week, I understood better the term "ambulance chasers."

I found the idea of hiring an attorney somewhat unsavory. I had no intention of suing the woman who hit me. I did not expect a financial windfall that would whisk me away to easy street. I simply wanted to get back to the moment before the crash—in my own little car, my own little job, my own little life. And since I was covered by a car insurance policy, a home insurance policy and insurance from my employer, retaining an attorney seemed a little distasteful and a lot redundant.

The word "naïve" comes to mind.

It would be 188 days before my auto insurance company would accept responsibility for paying wage-loss benefits and providing me with transportation to my countless appointments. Think about that. Think about all the times you barely make it to payday. For almost seven months I was forced to max out credit cards, take cabs or hope friends could drive me everywhere, and rely on my parents' generosity to save my house and keep me from slipping under the tidal wave of incoming bills. My friends basically fed my animals and me. I don't know what I would have done if I had been the sole breadwinner of a family with (human) children.

The accident itself caused trauma serious enough to generate ripple effects for years to come. The wrenching experience of going from quiet, working, bill-paying citizen to accident-victim in the eyes of insurance companies and the government carried similar long-term repercussions. My friend Roberta introduced me to attorneys Simkins & Simkins, PC. They are a well-respected firm actively involved in the Brain Injury Association of Michigan. The fact that they specialized in brain injury was vital. They were seasoned veterans in a game I had no idea I was even suiting up for. Looking back, the idea of heading into battle without them would be like trying to use a squirt gun to fight a tank battalion. There is simply too much we civilians don't know.

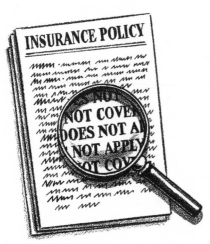

If you think "full coverage" promises blanket insurance against all catastrophes large and small, then you believe as I did, and you are in trouble. I paid sizable premiums to obtain coverage that I felt was more than adequate, and was comfortable in that security. After the accident, I was thrust into a system that had no intention of wrapping me in a fuzzy woolen blanket and making me a cup of warm milk. I found that I was only the recipient of familial welcome when I was paying my premiums. The welcome evaporated when I needed to use the benefits I had paid for.

I don't begrudge insurance companies their practice of using adjusters to minimize costs. These people have a job to do and that job is to minimize payouts. They're hired to say no. But when you suffer a brain injury, or any injury, your priority should be getting well and returning to life, not looking through the lining of your winter coats for change to buy tampons.

My attorneys did more than secure benefits for me to live on. They also offered the extraordinary value of their experience in the head injury community. They were tirelessly patient, and willing to address questions and concerns from my entire family. They listened to my frustrations as the blinders came off and I found myself questioning the medical/insurance system. Often, tests and X-rays do not conclusively isolate

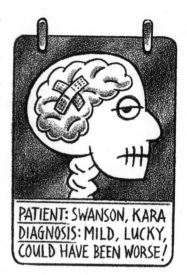

PATIENT: SWANSON, KARA
DIAGNOSIS: MILD, LUCKY, COULD HAVE BEEN WORSE!

major damage. Proving you are really injured, and not faking symptoms to extend a medical leave of absence, can be absolutely agonizing—and even more difficult when the injury is deemed "mild."

I must take a moment here to mention "malingering." I was first made aware of the term while reading articles and journals by leading professionals regarding head injury recovery. It seems that in the absence of conclusive results regarding recoveries—or lack thereof—in some cases, the authors were inclined to offer the possibility that some victims of brain injury were simply *choosing not to recover* more fully.

I cannot adequately describe to you how it feels to lose the life you have known. I cannot tell you exactly how it feels to look at part of your body and realize that it no longer takes commands from you. I cannot explain the frustration that comes with *not* healing, not recovering everything, not reclaiming your entire life. I cannot imagine anyone choosing to portray this kind of injury where it doesn't exist. I cannot imagine anyone staying on the bus long past their stop simply because they think the view is spectacular. We're talking "unfathomable" here.

I used to wonder why elderly people were often so stubborn in their refusal to surrender their driving privileges. We've all been frustrated by someone who can barely see over the steering wheel puttering along in the passing lane. Yes, I support the need to make sure people aren't dangerous to themselves or others. But how we take for granted the simple status of independence! And now I know why people fight so hard to keep it.

I know full well that there are those who deceive the government in order to keep receiving Social Security Disability or other government benefits in lieu of working an honest job. And I understand that it is the rightful responsibility of insurance companies and government agencies to contend with those who make it difficult to take truthful people at their word.

But I'll tell you what: I know of no benefit great enough to inspire relinquishing one's self-esteem and freedom of choice. Governmental assistance isn't the goal. For me, accepting Social Security Disability would mean giving up more than $20,000 of the annual income I was used to. Would I *choose* that? Would I perpetuate a tale that might eventually find me homeless, unemployable, and with a ruined credit history? Would I cut myself off from so many of the things I enjoyed for the privilege of living on $847 a month? *Come on!*

The feeling of earning a paycheck and being able to take care of the financial obligations in one's life is another satisfaction most people take for granted. But no one should.

My recovery and attempts to keep the injury from consuming my life were made vastly more difficult by the ridiculous need to prove I was injured. I had to undergo what seemed like a never-ending series of medical exams, conducted by doctors working for insurance companies and the government, to see if I was really hurt. I was scrutinized and evaluated and made to feel like a criminal.

I was asked the same questions over and over. Sometimes they would let me start over or give me hints when I asked. After half a dozen repetitions, I started offering more creative answers. When they asked me to name presidents, I would choose Taft or Hamilton—anyone but Clinton, Reagan or Kennedy. Or I would ask them if they wanted presidents of all the Fortune 500 companies I could think of, or of major league baseball franchises. They would ask me what was similar about a tree and a bush, and I would tell them they had the same number of letters in the word. By the fifth time through, even with my memory problems, I knew the answers.

Refusing to pad my symptoms for the benefit of those conducting evaluations put me in the unexpected predicament of possibly sacrificing my future financial security for what was left of my integrity. Finally, although I had heard horror stories of doctors proclaiming even the most severely injured to be well enough to return to work, my injury was confirmed without my having to compromise my ethics or put on an act.

Given that yes, I did have brain damage, I guess I was fortunate they concluded that yes, I did have brain damage. *Yippee skippee.*

Insurance laws vary from state to state. I live in Michigan, where our no-fault law encourages all drivers to carry insurance by making coverage affordable for practically everyone. It's also designed to eliminate complex determinations of accountability in accidents that might give birth to lengthy and sizable lawsuits. It outlines medical coverage for victims, structures liability parameters, and caps settlement ceilings.

In my case, it probably wouldn't have mattered whether I had died or merely suffered a scraped knee. The law requires that drivers carry only a minimal amount of liability insurance, in case they are found at fault in an accident. And I sure wasn't hit by Bill Gates.

Because I was under the impression that I was so fully insurance-covered, I didn't read the fine print of my policies until after my accident. Foolish me! I later found out that for pennies more a day, I could have secured coverage on my homeowners' policy that would have kept me floating above poverty in the event I became disabled. Instead, I found that I was covered if a golf cart accident happened on my property. How useful.

I also found out that my auto insurance carrier could have provided me with critical additional insurance benefits called "underinsured motorist" coverage. It's not promoted or made readily available to the vast majority of drivers. Had I known it existed, or known enough to apply for it, I would have been able to save my home and take care of my financial obligations with little worry. Not many of the big-name companies even offer "underinsured motorist" coverage. The bummer for me was that mine did, and I didn't have it.

My advice to everyone is to *read your policies*. Right now, before you leave your house again. Right now, before the unexpected happens. Insurance is money in the bank, medicine in the cabinet, doctors by the bedside, and hope on the horizon. Insurance is more than an expensive obligation; it's an invaluable opportunity to ensure that, should something horrific happen to us or to our loved ones, we do not risk losing everything in the process.

But no matter what your insurance coverage is, attorneys trained and specializing in brain injury are vital. Accident survivors are overwhelmed with the medical side of recovery, and often cannot fully participate in securing the benefits due them after injury. Even if they are physically capable of seeking benefits and filling out the awesome mountain of paperwork, they simply have no idea what's involved.

My case never went to court. I appeared at a deposition hearing 10 months after the accident to offer my account of the incident and its aftermath. By that time, the woman who had rammed into me had gone from blaming me for the accident (her position in April) to not being able to speak English and needing a translator (her assertion in November). "Wow!" I thought. She wasn't hurt in the accident she caused, but son of a gun, she had worse symptoms than I did. I merely stumbled over my words. She lost the entire English language.

The attorney for the woman who hit me was refreshingly compassionate. Her integrity was a welcome surprise in what I had anticipated would be a grueling experience. She offered to settle for the meager amount of insurance the liable driver carried, and with it, I was able to bring current some credit cards and prepare to sell the home I could no longer afford. However, in order to receive the settlement, I had to sign a document that would effectively close the case, release her of any future responsibility and exonerate her of all liability. Perfect.

The decision not to sue and try for a larger and fairer settlement was an agonizing one. There's no way to noodle through all the complexities involved without competent legal counsel. My counsel advised me that the laws in Michigan don't always smile warmly on people in my situation. If

I had gone to court and lost, I would have been potentially liable for paying the other side's legal fees and costs. I would have forfeited the settlement money and the insurance coverage for my lost wages. I wouldn't have received the cash I so desperately needed at the time we settled, and God knows how long it would have taken to fight through to victory even if we did eventually win. And I was always conscious of how hard I had heard it was to *prove* a closed head brain injury—especially a "mild" one—to a jury who probably understood nothing about the issues involved.

Before my accident I lived in a world that I thought honored its commitments and followed the law. I also thought that laws were made to protect and assist victims of criminal action. I was too ignorant to comprehend how ugly and tangled our system can be. Survivors and their families must vigorously pursue all possible avenues to have any chance of not being ruined by that system after a tragic injury. Seeking out qualified, respected law firms that deal exclusively or predominantly with the specific injury one has suffered must be a top priority.

Closing Wounds
With Red Tape

DR. DO-LITTLES

June 27, 1996

I wonder if I get frequent flyer miles. I think I should at least be getting free scrubs by now or bonus coupons for the cafeteria. I've been to these hospitals so many times that I'm starting to know everyone by name.

August 30, 1996

One of Dr. Cini's assistants asked me if I wanted "my room" redecorated.

My next book is going to be a coffee table picture collection of Michigan's finest hospital cafeterias. I will reveal where you can find the best coffee, the freshest Tootsie Rolls and the most comfortable chairs.

One of the reasons a head trauma survivor becomes so all-consumed with the recovery process is that there is little time for anything else. I was totally unaware how exhaustive the diagnostic and rehabilitative course becomes for someone who has sustained such an injury.

I'm very fortunate. Dr. Cini gave me the opportunity to undergo treatment wherever it was best provided. She deferred to specialists for many of my problems and, in this new world of managed health care and the stranglehold it is perceived to have on our doctors, I was afforded some of the finest professionals Michigan has to offer. Not to mention the Tootsie Rolls.

If you visit your doctor just once a year for a flu shot, you might not notice how frustrating the system can be. But when extended care is required, it becomes obvious how easy it is to get lost in the simple wish to be well again.

Every time Dr. Cini ordered a test, consultation or service, she was required to prepare a referral to be approved or declined by my health insurance carrier. After an approval was sent to my home, I would then make the appointment and receive the treatment. Simple enough, no?

Because I was injured in a car accident, my auto insurance carrier eventually assumed responsibility for paying the medical bills. My doctor would still have to fill out a referral for my health insurance because the auto carrier required that all treatment be "deemed necessary" and a written account be made available. The health insurance carrier would automatically decline it and it would then be forwarded to the auto insurance company. Even though Michigan does not require its auto carriers to preauthorize payment for services rendered, most of my treating facilities wanted to check first to make sure they would eventually be paid. Can't really blame them for that.

Depending on how quickly the referrals were being pushed through my doctor's office, the health insurance company and the auto carrier, the approvals would show up at the door anywhere from two weeks to two months after they were first requested. Imagine the weeks of waiting involved when I was referred separately for a neurological evaluation, a physiatrist who ordered two MRIs and monthly follow-up visits, a CT scan of the brain, a PET scan of the frontal lobe, physical/speech/occupational therapies, vestibular testing and retraining that led to hearing tests, neuro-optical field scans, driver's retraining and alternative-vocational therapy. You begin to understand the meaning of "diagnostic process."

Among the unsung heroes in my journey were the drivers from Give-A-Lift who took me to my appointments as a covered benefit. Those drivers, as well as all the technicians, physician's assistants, nurses and administrative people tried to answer all of my questions (especially in the beginning, when it is safe to assume I was a pain in the ass) and managed to keep my spirits up most of the time. They were big-time contributors to my understanding of how many genuinely good people are out there working for us to get well.

But I saw the other side of the system, too. As much as you may come to appreciate the efficiency and care afforded by competent doctors and professionals, you also become terribly *in*tolerant of those who lack respect for their patients and their patients' time. There weren't that many, but a few of the doctors I saw consistently took 45 minutes to an hour, sometimes longer, to get to their patients. One therapist told me everything about her life, her marriage, her kids and her own physical problems before our third session together. I knew the intimate details of her hysterectomy on my first visit.

One of my doctors told me that, although I showed no improvement after six weeks in his care, he *had* to report my therapy as "successful." I told him that I was no better off and knew nothing more than before seeing him, and he told me that he simply *cannot* put "that sort of thing" in his reports. For my alternative-vocational therapy, I waited more than eight months from referral to first visit, and that delay was attributed to the very people who were supposed to be trying to help me return to work. Amazing.

Our system sets up its medical professionals to work in an environment that is pressure-packed and quota-oriented. It leaves them little time to afford their patients consistently premium care. Having Dr. Cini quarterbacking my team enabled me to distance myself from the occasions of subpar treatment and lack of professionalism. I have seen her over 30 times since my accident. She and her staff remain consistent reminders of how the medical side of recovery can be run with efficiency, filled with compassion and spiced with humor.

"Not Tonight, Honey, I Have a Headache"

UNDERSTANDING THE SURVIVOR

August 29, 1996

They will find me in yesterday's pajamas. In yesterday's hair. In yesterday's makeup. And I will not care. I slept from 4 PM to 7 PM, then went to bed at midnight. I was wide awake at 4 AM, eating Spaghetti-Os and doing laundry. I went back to bed at 8 AM and slept till 1:30. I never know if I'm actually going to bed or just taking a nap. I'm starting to take after my cat ...

September 3, 1996

I have now organized, categorized and alphabetized my pantry. All of my linens are arranged by color and size and they all face the same way. I have color-coded my hangers to match my suits. I take more time picking out the pattern of my paper towels than I did buying this house. Even my Lazy Susan is efficient. Man, I really need to get a life.

Maybe people who tell their partners they don't want sex because they have a headache (every night) are really suffering from closed head injuries ...

I'm no medical doctor, although I watch *ER* faithfully. (Sometimes I diagnose the other patients in my doctors' waiting rooms, but I'm not sure that counts.) Still, I know there is a decided difference between feeling depressed sometimes and suffering from depression. There is a decided difference between feeling tired sometimes and suffering from fatigue. And there is a decided difference between having the occasional stress headache and suffering from traumatic head pain.

Although head injuries are particular to each survivor, common symptoms include the subtle, nagging sensation of "not feeling right." Many people suffer headaches relentlessly and are often medicated for them. Sleep patterns are likely disturbed. The dangerous combination of not understanding the injury, the length of the recovery process, and the damage to cognitive and physical abilities catapults brain injury victims to the top of the depression-watch list. And the very nature of the injury itself renders most survivors daily casualties of mental and physical fatigue. I'm not talking cuddly, sleepy-night-night, nappy-land tired here. No. I'm talking the kind of creature that creeps up and captures mind and body, submerging them in gooey oatmeal. And trying to explain these symptoms or find understanding for them is one of the most frustrating problems of all.

I had headaches. I have them still. It took a long time for them to settle into a pattern and potency that I could manage, tolerate and anticipate through medication and activity. They have been reduced from one of the most painful and difficult initial aspects of my injury to a calculated, daily annoyance.

A lot of people can understand chronic head pain, especially if they suffer from migraines or have endured severe allergies. It makes you less active, less talkative, less efficient and very grumpy. The fatigue factor is a little more difficult for people to understand. I'm sure they must think, "How can you be so tired when you don't work anymore?" Or, "You think *you're* tired, try working full time and having kids!" The only thing I can compare it to might be the feeling people get when they suffer from sugar-level dysfunction. They know what it's like to hit bottom after a sugar high and know they will soon be out for the count, whether they're ready with their footie-pajamas on or not.

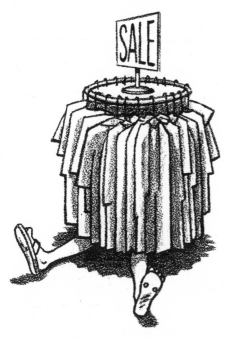

Ah, the places I have slept. When I first started driving again, I could get to most of the places I wanted to go, but couldn't make it back without needing to sleep. I would pull the car over, anywhere, and nap until I was rejuvenated enough to get home. Sometimes I would simply try to do too much in an outing. Once, two nice ladies woke me up under a clearance rack in the back of a Target store. When I'm going down, it doesn't much matter where.

Try to picture your body being managed by a little person inside your brain. She comes out and stands on a box and speaks into a microphone. She designates jobs, assigns tasks, gives directions and initiates commands to the entire body. As soon as she speaks, her messengers take off to all parts of the body with lightning-quick speed. They deliver the commands and messages and directions in less than split seconds to ports all over the body, manned by trained personnel waiting to receive word and follow orders. You walk, you reach, you speak, you smile ...

When someone suffers a brain injury, picture that inner person throwing her computer against the wall (which, by the way, in a snit I have done). Or picture her trying to organize and manage the entire fleet of messengers after drinking a bottle of tequila. Maybe she gets the orders wrong. Maybe she's onstage doing karaoke with a lampshade on her head. (Oh yeah, that was me *before* the accident.) Maybe the messengers themselves are drunk and mistake the information. Maybe they are staggering and cannot get to the ports as quickly as before. And maybe the people manning the ports are in the back room playing poker and smoking cigars.

In other words, picture anything that helps you imagine the myriad ways the components of an incredibly complex process—the human nervous system—can enter a state of fatal distraction.

Because the brain is so complex and so efficient, it immediately targets problem areas and begins to fix them itself. Some of the damage is corrected through the natural process of healing. For example, initial blindness might correct itself when pressure on the brain due to swelling recedes. Working systems around the damaged area might recognize they need to help out or fill in, and inherit that function or adapt compensatory techniques to improve its productivity.

In my case, the seat belt held my body still while the impact sent my brain smashing against the right side of my skull. All of a sudden, the little person on the box is processing foreign signals and confusing information. She has to assess the damage and find new personnel to fill in where others quit or were fired. She has to train these new people to work a system that is not functioning properly. And, she has to do it with the equivalent of a tequila hangover. The poor gal is exhausted.

Brain-injured people work twice and three times as hard to do half the work their brains did before. Whereas "normal" people walk into a restaurant and, with the speed of a computer, know immediately where the carpet ends and the tile floor starts and where the rest rooms are and where the screaming kids are seated, the brain-injured person is processing that same information with the speed of a pocket calculator. And, late in the day, the batteries in the pocket calculator run low on juice. Put it this way: the Energizer Bunny clearly does not have a head injury.

Eventually, proper rest and periodic downtime become as essential to most brain-injured people as insulin is to the diabetic. Successful recovery is about realizing what now works—because of what now *doesn't* work. And for helpers and supporters, recovery is about knowing that the survivor is the same person, but realizing that he has to rebuild parts of himself and his life.

A brain injury survivor might very well *look* and *sound* about the same as before the trauma. That complicates the challenge of understanding what's going on behind the scenes—and behind the forehead—and properly setting the bar of expectation. In this chapter I wanted to emphasize some of the common problems facing survivors, and fatigue is one of the most prominent. Families, friends, doctors and therapists must all have a shared understanding of the individual they're helping through this difficulty.

As for the dilemma of "Not tonight, honey, I have a headache," well, my therapist also works as a couples' counselor.

Spit and Vinegar

HEAD AND SHOULDERS ABOVE THE REST

May 13, 1997

Sometimes I want to scream. I look at people who stand nearer to this bus than they would ever want to imagine, and I want them to see me, pressing my face against the window. It's like salt in the wound when someone I know drives without a seat belt or won't wear a helmet. I just want to shake 'em and say, LOOK! Look at me!

I won't pretend to be an expert in anything but my own experience, and the logical and considerable lessons I have taken from it. And I don't want to come across as a holier-than-thou, pious hypocrite who thinks she now has the right to tell everyone how to live. But I won't stop hoping that nobody else gets on this damn bus. It's crowded here. And we're not exactly singing camp songs. Simply put: if you're not on it, you're not invited. Trust me, you don't want the ride.

Recent statistics on head injury from the Brain Injury Association are somber reminders that we have a long way to go to improve our safety. Consider:

- Every 16 seconds a head injury occurs in the United States.

- 140,000 persons die annually from head injuries.

- Head injuries are the number one killer of Americans under the age of 44. They kill more of us under the age of 34 than *all diseases combined.*

- Head injuries account for 500,000 hospitalizations each year.

- Two-thirds of all persons sustaining head injuries are under the age of 30. Young men are more than twice as likely as women to suffer head injury.

- Only 1 survivor in 20 is receiving appropriate rehabilitation today.

- One million children sustain a head injury each year. About 165,000 will be hospitalized, and 1 in 10 will suffer moderate to severe impairments.

Only in the last few years have we really begun to get the message across that seat belts save lives and that helmets are critical for bikers and skaters. It wasn't long ago that National Hockey League players weren't even required to wear a helmet—and many didn't. Even with 300,000 head injuries occurring in sports each year, the last of the helmetless hockey players only recently retired. Given how frequently it occurs, people should be as knowledgeable about the health hazard of head injury as they are about the flu.

Part of the problem is that our society tends to wait until there is a familiar face linked to a particular cause. Rock Hudson changed the face of AIDS. Gilda Radner made us more aware of ovarian cancer. Christopher Reeve is bringing national attention to spinal cord injury.

Professional—even collegiate—athletes are encouraged and expected to play with pain. The saying, "No blood, no foul" goes way beyond the playing surface, back into the training rooms. Because a head injury does not always boast blood and gore, it often goes undetected or disregarded. When there are championships and millions of dollars at stake, players who play with pain are also going to be inclined to play with a headache, a little dizziness, and the feeling of "being off." Every time I see another NFL quarterback return to football after a concussion, I cringe. It's a wonder that serious or multiple head injury isn't more prevalent.

As our understanding of the complexity of the brain grows, we know more and more what an incredible machine we have working for us. It would seem that something so precious, so vital, would command more of our attention and more of our effort to preserve it in working order.

But it doesn't. Face it, we live our lives with reckless abandon. I'm not just talking about young people who are full of the "nothing can happen to me" bravado of youth we all go through. I'm talking about everyone who takes his or her sound mind for granted. I'm talking about everyone who still refuses to wear a seat belt. Or the people who get drunk and climb behind the wheel of a car and put it into motion.

My friends, take it from someone who has had to watch her body and her mind refuse her commands. Do the right things to assure your safety. Take nothing for granted! Don't assume it can't happen to you. Hell, I wore my seat belt. I drove within the speed limit. I was not drunk. I did nothing reckless. It didn't matter.

My brain is damaged.

Even though I don't recall the morning of my accident, I know I didn't wake up and think, "Today my life will change forever." Nobody goes off to work or school thinking they won't come home in the same condition, or that they won't come home at all. Nobody calls everyone they love every morning and says their final good-byes because they figure they're about to die. You never know when your life is going to change forever. Don't tempt disaster by refusing to take the simplest measures to avoid it.

Kids are out on bikes and skates without helmets because they think helmets aren't cool. Teens aren't wearing seat belts because they are trying to pack eight friends in the car to go cruising on Friday nights. People are working in their homes and at their jobs in unsafe conditions because they are too lazy or too ignorant to wear protective gear. Drivers are putting on makeup, shaving, talking on cell phones, turning around and screaming at their kids. They spend more time trying to find a radio station than it would take to buckle their seat belts 10 times over. I don't get it.

Somebody told me recently they caught themselves not buckling up and they thought, "Geez, Kara would kill me!" Well, I'm not the one to worry about. It's the person flying out of a parking spot or running the red light who is going to kill you! I am delighted so many people have told me my accident has inspired them to wear their seat belts, but I want them to do it for *themselves*, for *their* safety, not because I'll chew on them if I find out they didn't.

Think about the odds we've all played, then thank your lucky stars for the times you've driven drunk and not killed yourself or someone else. Knock on wood for the time you fell off your bike without a helmet on and only scraped your knee. Count your blessings that the accident two seconds after you passed through that intersection not wearing a seat belt didn't have your name written on it.

And then get smart.

Head injury is a lot easier to prevent than to cure. There's no vaccine to resist it. There are no magic pills to destroy it.

There is only information, precaution, common sense and safety equipment. And even then there are no guarantees.

Tough as it's been to live with and recover from my injury, I'd rather be the one who was hit than the one who injured an innocent someone else. I don't envy anyone who has to live with the fact that they could have prevented an accident to themselves, their children, someone they loved— or even a total stranger, for that matter—because they did or didn't do something.

I also cringe at the memory of how many accidents I could have caused myself. I've juggled lunch on the run or struggled to take my coat off while driving. I have driven with four roaming kittens trying to crawl under my gas pedal. I drove drunk when I was ignorant and foolish. I played tag running along the tops of slippery poolsides when I was a kid. I don't think they even made helmets for us to wear while roller skating back then. If they did, no one knew enough to insist we wear them. We didn't know any better then and many of us were simply lucky. We no longer have that excuse, and hundreds of thousands of innocent victims will tell you all you care to hear about depending on luck.

Even now, when I know better, sometimes I still allow obstinate pride to stand in the way of my own safety. Maybe not when I drive, or when I'm responsible for someone else's safety, but sometimes I want *so badly* to do the things I used to do. I want to walk upstairs, for heaven's sake! Simple things that are no longer simple. I understand my reasons for wanting to do foolish, unsafe things. And they're poor, and I have to resist them, and everyone else needs to resist their reasons for being foolish and unsafe, too. If the bus drives by you without stopping, don't go chasing after it, waving your arms and calling it back. Times change.

Remember when condoms were considered "uncool"? People were embarrassed to buy them and hesitant to discuss them with their partners. We hid them behind the counters in drugstores. Well, safe sex is "in," gang! *Not* wearing a condom and *not* talking about safe sex and *not* protecting yourself is uncool now. Hint.

Please don't let your kids ride their bikes without helmets. Set a positive example that might save their lives one day ... and maybe yours in the process. And wear your own helmet on that family outing. What will you have accomplished by leaving your healthy child without a healthy parent? If you're driving, wear a seat belt. If you're drunk, don't you dare get behind that wheel. We are too aware and have too much information available to make excuses for our behavior. Some decisions are indefensible and we know it.

If you don't wear a helmet because it musses your hair or you don't buckle your seat belt because you think it's uncool, imagine how you'll look when someone is changing your diapers for the rest of your life. Or who will care how your hair looks when you're sitting at the table shoving mashed peas into the side of your face. I've seen it. There's nothing cool about it.

You have to love and respect yourself, your future and your potential. You have to prioritize those irreplaceable elements of yourself. You can't sacrifice them at the altar of momentary superficiality. You can always iron the seat belt wrinkle out of your shirt. You can't iron a wrinkle out of your brain.

Please, take "Kara" yourselves.

Halftime

WATCH WHAT YOU WISH FOR

I have my books
And my poetry to protect me
I am shielded in my armor
Hiding in my room
Safe within my womb
I touch no one and no one touches me
I am a rock
I am an island

—Paul Simon

September 11, 1996

Something has to change, Kara. The world stands still here and you do, too. Life has stopped and you have to find the energy and the inspiration somehow to rejoin it. My God, you don't even get dressed anymore! You don't take care of yourself. You sidestep invitations and you have become so isolated.

Halftime lasts 20 minutes for a college basketball game. How long should it last for a life?

I was a coach for many years before my accident. I coached basketball and softball and helped run summer camps for kids. I even had the opportunity to accompany a group of some of the best high school athletes from the Midwest to Australia to introduce Americanized volleyball there.

One of the most important aspects of coaching is game preparation. But it is not *the* most important. Coaches watch films of opposing teams. They target plays and propose counterattacks designed to keep opponents from executing their strategies. They run their teams through seemingly endless drills and scrimmages, and tutor them on fundamentals, sportsmanship and team play.

All that is fine and dandy. But what propels an ordinary coach to the status of a Bo Schembechler or a Chuck Daly or a Scotty Bowman is not only how well they prepare to go into a game. It is how they react and what they do when their opponent has scored the first three times down the field, or fired the first two shots into the back of the net, and things aren't working, and it's time for Plan B.

It is intermission. It is halftime.

A good coach will know there are holes in the secondary, or the back door is open, or the low-post is weak. He will know they are giving up the puck in the neutral zone or if the other goalie is open "top shelf." A good coach can take his or her team into the locker room and determine what needs to be changed. Maybe he'll ignite their competitiveness with fiery speeches. Perhaps he'll calm them down and quietly feed their confidence. The effective coach provides them with ways and means to bounce back and produce. His team will come back on the field or the rink or the court ready to fight again, ready to shrug off frustration, ready to implement logical options to improve performance.

After the Detroit Red Wings trounced the National Hockey League record for regular-season victories in '96, they fell surprisingly in the playoffs. Many people were flabbergasted when, in the off season, they significantly retooled a roster thought to be inches from a Stanley Cup. Scotty Bowman took much of the heat for trimming the squad of several fan favorites. He acted boldly. He brought in the likes of Brendan Shanahan and Larry Murphy from other teams. He gave more responsibility to Nick Lidstrom, Darren McCarty and Martin Lapointe. He mixed a surprising bag of veterans and rookies that would jeopardize his reputed genius if the '97 run stalled.

He was a good coach. He was not going to sit idle and allow his team to repeat the debacle of being swept by the New Jersey Devils in the '95 finals or the '96 stunning at the hands of the Colorado Avalanche. He was giving his team a legitimate shot. He was saying that what they were doing was not working quite well enough, and no matter how difficult the decisions, they had to be made.

Well, I thought I was a good coach. Until the game was *my* game, my life.

Those first months were, NBA-metaphorically, like getting full-court pressed with no point guards to bring the ball up. They were like looking down the bench and seeing all seven-foot centers who had never learned to dribble. I had no one who could come in and take command of the ball and the offense. I was flailing.

Ginger kept after me. She insistently prodded me to not wait passively for this period of injury to end, to not wait (continuing the NBA metaphor) for Joe Dumars to come through the locker room door, change into uniform and take charge of my offense. I so wanted Dr. Cini or someone to look me straight in the eye and tell me, "OK, Kara, we've done everything we can. Now go off and restart your life. Here's what you need, here's a list of what you can do, here's where to go and who to call." I wanted the "New Life Starter Kit." I was looking for someone or something to take control of the offense and it took me a long time to realize that I *was* the offense.

If you believe in capital-F Fate, you comfort yourself with the understanding that everything happens for a reason. Sometimes those reasons are merely rationalizations that allow us to accept the unfathomable. I embrace the Fate theory, especially when tragic events occur that are so horrific that I have no other way to process them: a child who dies from a rare disease; a person who goes happily into a bank to cash a check and gets shot during a holdup; a plane full of passengers lost when a malfunction sends a jet down into the Atlantic. Sometimes there are no answers, no logic. But part of our human makeup is that we need to know *why*. We crave reasons for the things that happen. When reasons aren't available, the only straw to cling to may be the concept of Fate.

Before my accident, I basically lived for my work. My 13-year career often demanded 18-hour days and 7-day weeks. I worked holidays and weekends. Work was not a part of my life; life was a part of my work. And a small one at that.

I always thought that one day I'd write a book. The image of that future accomplishment was comforting. Somehow, I'd find the time to create the novel hidden inside me. As I wrote, I would look out the window of an old Victorian farmhouse on a lake that would inspire great thoughts and serene wisdom. That was the dream.

I hadn't written anything yet because people always said, "Write what you know and what is true," and I couldn't think of any truths I knew that might be important enough for people to read. I was a caterer; I figured people already knew how to eat. And I didn't have the time to take my clothes to the cleaners, much less sit down and write the Great American Novel. Writing was best left to the indefinite future, it seemed, to a time when I would be more witty, more wise, more mature, and less swamped with catering events.

Maybe I missed some signs along the way. Maybe Fate was whispering in my ear to change careers, embrace life, make time and find time. To commit myself to writing, commit myself to living.

If so, I didn't listen. So maybe my accident was Fate's way of shouting after I turned a deaf ear to its whispers. The accident took away my ability to work in my field, and it took away my ability to drive. It took away my endurance to work 18 hours a day. It took away my feet—but spared my hands. It took away my ability to say words, but not the ability to think them or type them. It stole much of my mobility and gave me all the downtime I could ever have wanted.

I am no longer swamped with catering orders. Watch what you wish for …

When Dr. Cini and Ginger suggested I write a book about recovering from brain injury, the irony was not lost on me. They were adamant about trying to get me to go into that locker room at halftime and make some adjustments, instead of coming out for the third quarter and continuing to get bombed.

I had written for Ginger before the accident, but I had to uncover those skills again, dig them out from the mental debris. I give her credit for having the wisdom to wait until she saw my writing ability return before she encouraged me to take it up seriously.

I didn't get off to a quick start. My first writing in the months immediately following the accident was bland and colorless. It was awkward and didn't come naturally.

But even after a little literary color came back, I had other challenges. My writing gamboled and hid from tradition and structure. Words ran rampant. I was once *so loyal* to grammar, sentence structure and punctuation. Now I was pouring out short, choppy thoughts and long, windy harangues. I was all over the place, a kite without a string, and no telling where I'd find myself next.

The inability to organize my thoughts confounded me. I had some idea of what I wanted to say, but I couldn't keep other ideas from popping in here and there, and my first few attempts were a tangled mess. The more I wrote, the more I confused the ideas. It was like trying to get gum out of my hair with mittens.

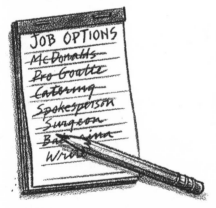

I so loved to write that I did not wish to find myself incapable of it. I couldn't bear the thought. I would rather not have tried than to try and fail at something I was once so proud of. I was scared.

I looked at other options for fulfillment. With my balance and reflexes, playing goalie for the Red Wings (or even the Black Hawks) was out. Brain surgery was also eliminated, as I tried to imagine putting Post-it notes on patients' heads to remember where each part went. With my inappropriate anger, most venues of public interaction were also eliminated. I could just imagine myself working the drive-through window at McDonald's and getting into a snit over something a customer said, or just having too many orders to fill. I'd be propelling Big Macs at customers in the parking lot! Then I looked at my weight and considered becoming a spokesperson for the new Grand Prix because, as they say, "Wider is better!"

When my occupational and vocational therapists asked me what I wanted to pursue now, I hesitated to tell them. Here I was, former caterer, newly brain-injured, telling these folks I wanted to write for a living. I could imagine their reaction. They would furrow their brows ever so slightly, put a hand on my shoulder, and tell me that maybe I should set my sights a little lower for the time being—maybe stick to something in the catering field (where I had spent my entire ca-*reer*, they would stress). They had already pointed out I could use a wheelchair at work, and suggested maybe my former employer could take me back a few hours a week doing something simple, like filing. It was logical. It was more dependable and more likely than what I was contemplating. It made sense at a time when I didn't have all that much confidence in myself. I wavered.

Without Dr. Cini and Ginger encouraging me to believe I could do more, I would likely have accepted a future of someone else's choosing. Halftime was over. I needed to commit to something.

I told Ginger I would need help until I got into a routine that felt comfortable. I sorely needed focus, so I asked her to assign me a certain number of pages to be written before each of our sessions. I gave her permission to figuratively kick my butt if I didn't have them done. And she did. I can laugh at that now. At the time, I didn't find her all that funny.

I could not get started. I couldn't concentrate. I couldn't focus on one idea and get it down on paper before getting sidetracked or losing interest. I would write for 45 minutes or so, then have to take a 3-hour nap. I would come back to the work and have no idea where I'd been heading with a particular topic or thought. Half the time I couldn't write the stupid sentences with what felt like 10 chubby thumbs, or read them bouncing back and forth on the paper.

After the first few chapters, I stopped persecuting myself for not being able to sort out topics and thoughts. (However, I *did* persecute myself for having two page 65s and misnumbering the last 40 pages.) The priority became not to write the next *Moby Dick,* but simply to write—and through that writing, to extend a hand to someone Fate had chosen to board the same bus I was riding. I felt that was worth a try.

The Thanksgiving holiday played a special part in the process. Without it, this book would never have gotten off the ground. When I was a kid, my mom cooked the greatest Thanksgiving Day meals. Some of my fondest memories are of that first wonderful smell of roast turkey wafting out of the kitchen, watching the Thanksgiving Day parade from downtown Detroit, and sneaking forkfuls of stuffing during the Lions games. My mom was a great cook, and on Thanksgiving Day she positively shone.

When Mom suffered disabling strokes in 1992, Thanksgiving Day became the elephant in the living room that none of us was ready to acknowledge. The idea of tying on my mother's apron strings was more frightening than the idea of cutting them off had ever been. Still, I cooked my first turkey that year, with both of us crying silently, not looking at each other. And with the easing and soothing that sometimes only time can bring to troubled situations, I have prepared our family's holiday feast every year since. It's an accomplishment that's become a source of great pride to me. A tradition has passed down from my mother to me, strengthening the bond between us.

I started thinking about the first Thanksgiving after my accident in early October. I wanted to do it. I wanted to succeed. Though everyone worried that it would be a day of frustration for me—and, quite possibly, a dismal failure—I declined their offers to take over my dinner preparation role.

During my career in food service I had learned to cook by the seat of my pants. I learned under wonderfully talented chefs who never prepared by recipe, always by creative imagination. But I knew I could no longer just skip into the kitchen and pull off a Martha Stewart soirée.

I scaled down the menu (out went the green bean casserole) and made an exhaustive supply list. Diana took me grocery shopping. When I asked her how many potatoes to get, she told me five. Anticipating the worst, I got nine. That would give me some backup units in case I had a snit and started throwing potato fastballs through the kitchen window.

I prepared each item the day *before* Thanksgiving. I didn't want to take a chance of ruining anything on the big day, so I cooked everything but the turkey. I figured, in effect, we would be having leftovers a day early. Everyone loves Turkey Day leftovers. I covered each pan, then labeled it to show its contents and how much it needed to be warmed the next day. After finishing each item, I completely cleaned my work area and sat down to rest so I wouldn't get frustrated or irky.

Thanksgiving Day arrived and so did my family. As they sat watching the Lions game, I forced myself to concentrate and focus, checking off items on my list as they finished cooking. The turkey was done an hour and a half earlier than I had expected. The biscuits had bottoms of charcoal and I forgot the milk in the au gratin potatoes. I was in bed for the next two days feeling like someone had dropped a tractor on my head. Still, some said it was the best Thanksgiving meal I had ever cooked. (I'm still thinking about the implications of that.)

That day I found something more than a marginal turkey dinner, something important that I had been searching for. It was the realization that I could succeed; that it might be difficult or different, but I could find a way, manage a way, to achieve the things I really wanted to do.

And something else happened that day. When we paused to give thanks for all that we were fortunate enough to have in our lives, I realized I had begun to *feel* something I knew intellectually. Something that used to drive me nuts when I heard others say it. That I *was* lucky. I *was* really fortunate. I was going to be able to come out for the second half after all.

Maybe my halftime speech to myself wouldn't be as fiery as one of Bo's. And maybe my writing wouldn't be as witty, intelligent and mature as it might have been had I waited for some future start date. But I realized the future was now, right there, carved to perfection on Mom's china platter. And I gave thanks.

Schooled

THE SUN ALSO RISES

February 3, 1996

Dianne, Kelly, Carolyn and Jessica drove 45 minutes just to bring me lunch and keep me company. Patti was going to come but she is sick so Ken showed up alone with flowers. Kim and Tracey are coming next week.

March 9, 1996

Tim and Ken are going to help get my house ready to sell as soon as the weather breaks. I can't believe it's really coming to this.

August 28, 1996

Sue comes tonight. She's flying in from California just to take me to my tests this week. These will be the grueling ones at U of M and she was thoughtful enough to come all this way ...

Yesterday I got a surprise package from Sari and Cindy in the mail. Today one came from Aunt Fredda. Neil brought lunch and Kris made spaghetti for dinner. What a great week!

I've often wondered: what lessons did I need to learn that made it necessary to go through all this? In deep, introspective moments I have sought the key message delivered via speeding minivan that crisp January morning. I figured that maybe if I hurried up, learned the lesson and absorbed the message, I would receive clearance to return to my old life. It was worth a try.

The roots of understanding and perspective grow from what we choose to keep, and how we slant the memory of events in our lives. It would have been easy—even understandable—for me to take the road to bitterness and resentment. I had that opportunity. And, admittedly, I dabbled.

I spent more time than I care to admit thinking "if" thoughts. If I had driven more slowly or more quickly ..if I had showered for one more minute ..if I had stopped for gas or taken that last sip of coffee ...Maybe then I would not have been in that intersection at that horrific moment.

The anger and resentment I had for the woman who hit me didn't solve any problems. If anything, it created more. It didn't bring back that morning. It didn't bring back my balance, my efficiency, my independence. Hating myself or cursing the circumstances that brought me into this predicament only wasted energy I needed to heal. I learned the hard way that as long as you stay in the past, you cannot have a future. No matter how hard it is, *you have to let go.*

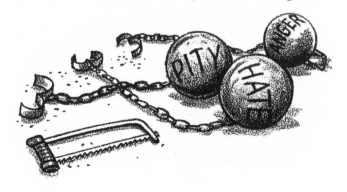

Even as I write those words, I continue to remind myself as well. It's a daily lesson, a moment's consideration that can affect an entire lifetime.

You can drive yourself crazy asking, "Why me?" or "What did I do to deserve this?" Worrying if we should leave earlier, stay later, take a different road, or book a later flight doesn't get us anywhere. We don't know what future awaits each course of action. In the end, there just aren't reasons for why some things happen. Not reasons we're allowed to see, anyway.

So instead of drowning in "what if," I try to be aware that some goodness has blossomed from the worst thing that ever happened to me. For one thing, I was forced to get out of a career that, in hindsight, was consuming my life. Only since the accident have I realized how much I was sacrificing for the job: family, friends, other interests. I was way out of balance. I'm still lacking balance, but now it's the straight-forward physical kind.

I see people in a different light now. Take cab drivers. Before my accident, cabs and cab drivers were an uninteresting, faceless mass of humans and machines that I didn't need. Suddenly, I couldn't drive. Now I needed them. When I first started calling them, all I did was whine and complain about how long it took to pick me up, how run-down their vehicles were, and how horribly they drove. But the anger was about me, not them. I so resented the fact that I could no longer drive that I directed anger at them. Once I accepted them and their services as a positive solution to my transportation problem, I found myself enjoying wonderful conversations with people who were bright and profound, witty and compassionate. They are some of the finest storytellers I've ever known.

I found out how ignorant I had been regarding differently abled people. I had been on the side of the fence with the healthy, the mobile, the able. I was not cognizant of the challenges people with disabilities face, the prejudice, the insensitivity, the misunderstanding. I was unaware of how little we, as a society, have made a safe and welcoming place for them.

Excuse me. For *us*.

Whenever I felt sorry for myself, something or someone came along with a much-needed dose of humility or insight. I remember when they first told me I would need to use a wheelchair. I was pretty self-pitying and sulky about it. While I was sitting on the couch boo-hooing my predicament and watching TV through sniffles and Kleenex, an unexpected show came over the cable: the Wheelchair Beauty Pageant. These women were pretty, talented and in great shape despite being in a wheelchair. They carried themselves with more class and dignity than I *ever* had. I was ashamed of myself.

Then there was the time I had a writing crisis. I couldn't find where I had saved one of my chapters in the computer. I didn't understand directory searches and structures (and still don't, as a matter of fact). All I understood was that I had misplaced something, couldn't find it, and was livid at being hammered once again by my new limitations. Then I read a story about a man who was stricken with a devastating illness that left him unable to move virtually any part of his body. He and a friend designed a code that would connect each letter of the alphabet with a certain number of *blinks*. Together, they wrote an entire book with the author blinking out each letter and each word. Compared to him, I had it all. Compared to him, I felt humbled and embarrassed that I would curse my situation. Timing is everything.

I am acutely aware of relationships that I wouldn't have had otherwise which were shaped and formed as a direct result of my injury. Some people go through their entire lives and never really know how many people care about them. I have been the recipient of a magnificent outpouring of kindness and generosity, and it swells my heart. Those first few days after my accident, my house was filled with plants and flowers and cards and calls. And they didn't stop.

People I had only known as work acquaintances became treasured friends. They sent me coloring books and surprise packages. They picked me up and took me out to dinner or shopping or just out of the house. People I barely knew were sending gift certificates for groceries, and offering prayers and hopes and silly jokes that took my mind off my troubles. My dentist's office called me once a month just to check up on me. My veterinarian sent a get-well card signed by her entire staff.

Friends contacted people they knew all over the country to find information that might help me. A knock at the door and Diana and Marty would come in with bags of groceries and dog food and cat litter. Rita would call to let me know there was food on my doorstep, dropped off by Mark or Justin while I was sleeping. I'd look out my window and see neighbors who barely knew me shoveling my snow or cutting my grass.

What did I learn from all this? Don't leave the important things unspoken. Don't leave the deep things unshared. We don't know how much opportunity for talking and sharing our futures hold for us. Maybe not enough to waste time and energy on issues and relationships that don't really matter. Maybe just enough to find, foster and cherish the ones that really do.

There are also people who shy away from me now. In a way I can't blame them. Hell, even I shied away from me for quite some time after the accident. It's hard—for them and for me. Those who remember me running down the court or sliding into third or coaching on the sidelines remind me of that person, too. The memories aren't lost. The images don't fade. Two-foot stop. Head fake. Up, release, follow-through, *swish!* That's who I was. That's who I chose to be.

Now, I'm a prickly and disquieting reminder that we don't have control over anywhere near as much as we think we do. That our lives don't follow a plan just because we make one. Maybe I'm the hand that smacks with the sting of reality. Very understandable if they see me that way. That's what I am for myself, every day.

I have restored and revived some relationships I was once too busy for, took for granted or didn't fully appreciate. I know my father better now and love him more dearly. I have an aunt in California who has become like a surrogate mother. I understand first-hand the problems my godfather has with his own balance dysfunction. I have new levels of old friendships so precious that I sometimes feel I would sustain this injury all over again to achieve them.

And I finally know a bit about humility. I look around me and find that my troubles often pale in comparison. There is always someone around the corner whose paths are rockier, valleys deeper, and nights colder.

I asked earlier what lesson I needed to learn, what cosmic purpose was being served here. Maybe that's it.

No, I don't wish this injury on anyone. Yes, it did end a life that was comfortable, successful and pretty enjoyable. But I am so very lucky to have a second chance. I learned important lessons that didn't demand death as payment. Many cannot say that. I have, finally, chosen to embrace this second life not as a consolation prize, not as a tragic sentence, but as a great gift. I may not be proud of how long it took me to get to this point. But I made it, and I'm grateful I didn't arrive too late.

A Seat on the Bus

NOTES FOR SURVIVORS

July 18, 1998

My face looks awful. There's something about the term "seeping pustules" that doesn't do much for my self-confidence. I've been using the cream Dr. Cini gave me so I don't keep waking up with my face covered in dried blood from scratching it in my sleep. This morning I got up and when I looked in the mirror, I scared myself half to death! The fan had blown loose dog fur during the night and it all stuck to the medicine on my face.

Well, this is rotten, isn't it?

I keep trying to think back and remember what it was that I wanted or needed to hear when I first had my injury. More than anything, I wanted something concrete to hang my hat on. (Instead, I got something concrete to *wear* my hat on.) I wanted the timetables they give you when you break your leg: six weeks in a cast with crutches, four weeks of physical therapy with crutches, maybe two with a cane, physical therapy, and then back to normal. It seemed that all I got were too many doctors saying they really didn't know when or how much I would heal. I've known parents who were less evasive when their kids asked them where babies came from.

Many people come back quickly from brain injury and suffer few, if any, residual effects. Their brains heal and they resume most or all of their normal activities within a few weeks or months. If you've ever been injured, I certainly hope you're one of them! Others, such as myself, will probably never quite get everything back. Ginger might have hit the mark when she told me I would have to wait for medical technology to catch up to me. She pointed out that every day we take exciting new steps toward better understanding the intricacies of the brain.

There's always hope! Sometimes you just have to look a little harder—or in peculiar places—to find it. Sometimes you have to take a realistic look at what it is you're hoping for. And sometimes all you can do is wait.

That last option is hard as hell.

Doctors can't give specific "heal dates" and promise exact outcomes, but they can make fairly sophisticated guesses based on the circumstances relating to your injury: how it happened, whether and where you suffered a direct body hit, whether—and for how long—you lost consciousness, and the symptoms you display. Different combinations suggest different degrees of damage. But even with the myriad possibilities, there are similarities and constants in head trauma that are likely to affect most survivors. Many can be helped with the same compensatory techniques or medication. If those don't help, knowing that so many others face similar challenges sometimes does.

As an injury survivor, one of the most important issues to assess immediately is your safety. You may be too impaired to recognize and understand all your symptoms. Impatience to get back to your normal life can put you in harm's way all over again. The people in your life, and your doctors, will attempt to ensure that your activities don't put you at additional risk. Be patient with them. They're only trying to help. When you are able to demonstrate logical, safe decision-making, they'll help you begin to reclaim your life and independence.

After that, it's a matter of tailoring your recovery to the unique features of your injury. A good doctor will make certain you have access to the best care. That means you will undergo more tests and schedule more appointments than you ever imagined you'd have in your whole life. And unfortunately, many of those tests will reveal more questions than answers. They're designed mostly to provide information that will assist in structuring optimized compensatory techniques for your rehab program. Sometimes—not often enough—tests will reveal that at least part of an injury can actually be repaired.

Try to remember that the doctors' prognosis is simply their best guess. You don't *have* to be defined by it or resigned to it. One of the best things about the brain is its magnificent ability to heal itself. And one of the best things about the human spirit is that, deep down, it wants the brain to try.

It's important to keep a journal about your activities and your progress. If you can't do it, ask a friend or family member. Get one of those daily calendars and keep track of what you did, what you experienced and how you felt each day. If you're unable to write, consider a tape recorder. Not only will it help your doctors, it will also assist in recalling details about such things as household services—who did what— that you'll need to report to your insurance provider. If your case ends up in court, it will help you more accurately complete the comprehensive interrogatories needed to prepare your case. And most importantly: it will be your own measuring stick of progress as you go forward.

From the moment you are diagnosed with a brain injury, you will find yourself besieged by paperwork. Depending on how you were injured and where, you may have forms from employers, hospitals, insurance companies, doctors and attorneys. There are probably entire categories of forms I never saw, but you might. I bought one of those folders that fan out like an accordion to hold them all and keep them organized.

Your body is going to exhaust itself trying to heal and you need to give it every opportunity. That makes plenty of sleep critically important. Early on, even the most basic activities may deplete your energy. You need to give yourself time to refuel.

Make things as easy as possible on yourself. If you are having problems with your memory, consider a whiteboard to keep track of your medications. You might buy a timer that counts down the minutes and hours to signal when you need to do something. It helps to have notepaper with you at all times, especially when you are with doctors who are providing important information regarding the next steps in your course of treatment. If you're having a difficult time with something, ask for help. Maybe someone can call to remind you to take your medication. (At one point, three of my friends were calling me at appointed times throughout the day to make sure I hadn't forgotten.) Do whatever works! Have friends come into your medical consultations with you so they can hear as well, and provide informed assistance if needed.

Information is the key. The more you have, the more you will understand exactly what your brain is doing—and *not* doing that it used to.

Headaches are a bummer. Unfortunately, most people who sustain brain injuries get them—and keep them for brutally long periods. The Incas used to treat their headaches by drilling holes in the offending skulls. (No market for Tylenol there.) I am thankful we've progressed, but I have to admit there were times when the pain was so awful that the Inca treatment didn't seem like a bad idea.

You need to create a place in your home that is conducive to reducing your head pain. This is not just a choice; it's something your body will demand. Many people find that it helps to go into a quiet room that is dark and cool. Loosen your clothing and close your eyes. Cold packs, heating pads, or a combination of both might help (you can find them in medical supply outlets). You don't want to mess with ice and water, especially if you have a heating pad. And electric heating pads aren't the greatest because they aren't safe if you are prone to falling asleep for long periods. Head injuries are not a death sentence—don't electrocute yourself! Try one of those pads you toss in the microwave for a minute or so.

The Brain Injury Association is a great source of information that will help you and the people in your life get through this (see p. 121 for BIA contact information). It operates chapters in many areas. They sponsor activities, send out newsletters, and support events and conferences planned to assist survivors and their families. Many attorneys and doctors belong to the association and may have pamphlets or flyers useful to you and the people helping you. All relevant information—whether from professionals or the waitress at Big Boy—can help. Collect it, share it, send it to your family and friends.

Your circumstances may or may not require consideration of a lawsuit, but either way, you should contact a law firm that specializes in head injury. Don't forfeit the opportunity to acquire needed legal representation because you think you can't afford it. Most of these legal specialists will arrange for a consultation when and where it is most convenient and comfortable for *you*. They will be up front about their fee structure and you will be relieved to discover that they make every effort to eliminate out-of-pocket costs.

I didn't have one, but many survivors enlist the services of "case managers." These people assist in all areas of recovery, from helping you fill out paperwork to following up on benefits or scheduling appointments. My attorneys and doctor took the role of case managers when my auto insurance declined the case manager I requested. From everything I hear, though, a competent case manager can help your recovery process maintain its momentum and stay its course.

Your doctor must be someone you feel comfortable with and trust. I was fortunate to end up with Dr. Cini, considering how I selected her. Like many people in this world of managed care, I picked her out of a catalog. I used a fine decision parameter, too: of the doctors' names in my area, I liked hers the best. By the time I was first introduced to her, she had gotten married and changed her name. It's a wonder we ever met, given my rigid qualifications! I didn't bother fully researching potential physicians because I figured I'd only be visiting her once a year, for a checkup or a flu shot. I never imagined I'd end up seeing her more often than I saw my parents.

Your doctor is your point person. He or she is going to lead and carry the flashlight as you head into the tunnel and make your way through dark, uncharted territory. You have to make sure that your doctor is going to take time with you and be available to you. You'll have questions. You'll feel frustration. You'll run into problems. That all demands time and attention. It won't work if your doctor doesn't connect with your personality, isn't compassionate, or knows little or nothing of head injury.

Carry information with you regarding your condition, medications, and physician's number in case you are in an emergency situation. Knowing that you already have a brain injury will help medical personnel adjust their initial tests if, God forbid, you find yourself facing another traumatic event. I wear a medallion around my neck with all my pertinent information. I carry an ID card and have sent emergency instructions to some of my close friends, including medications and the telephone numbers of my physician, therapist and attorney. I have also written a will and made some arrangements for my dogs and my cat. Maybe I'm overprepared, but that's better than being underprepared.

You're going to experience a lot of emotions, and they are all natural and expected. You may feel sad, angry and frustrated. You will find yourself impatient with the system and the length of your recovery process. Sometimes your progress will feel like you're crawling through maple syrup. Other times you'll glow with the tremendous satisfaction of demonstrable improvement.

If you don't heal right away, you'll lose facets of your life and you'll miss them. It might be your career or a favorite hobby. Maybe you won't be able to drive, or you'll lose your mobility. That translates to lost independence. Perhaps you have cognitive damage that has seemingly taken your wit, your organizational skills, your memory.

Whatever the injury has taken, you are certainly allowed to acknowledge that loss. While your family and friends will likely sympathize with your feelings, you may require additional help to adequately process and explore them. Though I'm no poster child for psychotherapy, I think it is one of the greatest elixirs available.

For a long time I was really hung up on the "moment my life changed" anthem. I could not get past it. I had purchased my first home shortly before my accident, moving across town to be near my new, better paying job. Then I found myself nose to nose with the front grill of a speeding minivan. I was far away from my family, most of my friends and the life I knew on the other side of town. My car was totaled. I had no real monetary nest egg. To keep me going financially and emotionally, my two bosses virtually adopted me.

I lost the opportunity to take on that new job. I lost my career. I could no longer afford the home I had just purchased. I missed a once-in-a-lifetime opportunity to work in Atlanta for the '96 Olympic Games. When it took seven months to sort out who was going to pay my lost wages, benefits and medical bills, I went into debt and needed money from my parents. I ruined my credit rating and jeopardized my ability to purchase another home or car. For the first time in my life I felt vulnerable, an easy target walking alone. My reputation in the catering business went from level head to lead head. Everywhere I looked, as far down the road as I could imagine, my injury continued to injure.

I had to realize that it didn't help to forever bemoan the moment my life changed. We change all the time. I changed every day before my accident, and I'll change every day after it. Change is not the problem. It is our inability or unwillingness to accept and recover from change that puts us most in jeopardy. Granted, expectations might not be fully met. We'll face curve balls when we were looking for sliders. But eventually, we just have to redefine "normal" and stop holding ourselves up to rules and expectations that no longer apply.

There isn't a single person I have met or read about who didn't eventually find some unexpected good coming into their lives as a result of their injury. Stories abound of positive aspects and outcomes found hiding in the wake of disaster. I was forced out of a career that, in retrospect, was effectively taking up my entire life. I understood better how my mother felt after two strokes took the life she was used to and left her with one she never intended. I am better able to commiserate with my father when he has trouble remembering little details or loses track of the date. Are these benefits worth the pain? No. But are they better than nothing? Absolutely.

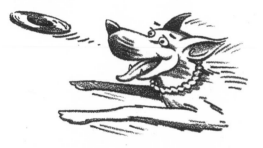

Animals can help in a patient's recovery. Research has consistently shown that animal companions reduce stress, anxiety and blood pressure in patients and the elderly. I was a stressed and anxious patient who sometimes felt a hundred years old. And my dogs and cat were up to the task.

They didn't care that I had growths on my face or that I was bumbling along with a cane. They loved and listened to everything I said, even when my words stuck and eluded me. They were gracious enough to get fat right along with me and, when I cried, their little eyes would get all squinty and they would lie right next to me, put their ears down and sigh. They were the first to remind me that I was still lovable, still the same person, still worthy of their wags and smiles. I would have been terribly lonely without them.

You *will* find your way. It will come to you. And if you don't find it, you will make one yourself. There are people out there trained, ready, available and anxious to help you survive with your sanity and self-esteem intact. Take advantage of their experience. Many of them have laid down their coats so you don't have to fall face-first into a mud puddle. No, your life may not be what it was before your injury. Even if you heal entirely, the experience will leave an indelible mark. But perhaps that won't be entirely bad. You may find that parts of the life you had before your injury were not all you imagined them to be.

You're going to have to make yourself a priority. You need to figure out who you really were before your injury in order to understand who you are now and who you might come to be. You'll probably be surprised at how different the world looks when the spectacles of perspective are more cracked than rose-colored. You might even find answers to questions you would not have thought to ask before you were hurt.

It's OK to do everything except lose hope, give up, throw in the towel. Recovery, you will find, is a life-long process.

But, my friend, anger and hatred will be nesting in you somewhere, and these feelings won't be easy to dislodge. Whether you feel partially responsible for your injury because of something you did or didn't do, or whether you hold someone or something else liable for it, those emotions are natural and expected. They are also destructive and dangerous.

You cannot change what has happened. No matter how hard you look at a picture, the images stay locked in the frame. Take that anger and that hatred and allow it, acknowledge it, voice it, recognize it and give it its moment. Then, for your sake, realize how important it is that you let it go. Understand the energy your body and brain need to heal, and do not waste it feeding something that seeks to consume you. Regardless of the circumstances that led you to the bus, fighting yourself promises only to lengthen your journey.

There are a lot of us, you know. More than you will ever first imagine. Too many. Some are worse off and some have it better. Some didn't make it at all.

We are a unique group. We don't care what circumstances brought you here. Nobody is less or more important. We're pulling for you! We're cheering you forward! We want you to hang in there, to survive and thrive, to find a life you can pursue, succeed in and enjoy.

Brain Injury Association
105 North Alfred Street
Alexandria, VA 22314
Family Help Line: (800) 444-6443
Phone: (703) 236-6000
Fax: (703) 236-6001
http://www.biausa.org

The Internet is a tremendously valuable source of information, products for the disabled, support groups and other resources. New web sites are added every day. Search under "brain injury" for a list.

Dear Family and Friends

A NOTE TO THE SUPPORT CREW

July 8, 1996

I hadn't slept for 56 hours. I finally called Dr. Cini and she prescribed something to help. Diana, Marty and Rita were here when I took it. I guess I was quite a project. Marty was standing behind me, mouthing to Diana not to leave me alone. Diana said I was telling her that the reason I walk the way I do is because I have no bones in my legs. I guess I did a couple of somersaults right off the side of the bed. I wondered why I am sore today. She stayed until I finally fell asleep. Safe. Lucky to have them.

Someone in your life has suffered a traumatic injury. Maybe your child, parent, spouse, friend, or a colleague at work. When you hear that someone has diabetes or cancer, you know immediately what that means. But the words "head injury" often don't have the same impact as a more familiar diagnosis. Maybe you know as much as I did—which is basically nothing—so you shrug. Or you are quick to fear the worst because you don't know enough, and apparently the doctors don't either.

Unfortunately, head injuries often mean you go on the "wait and see" list. Much of the patient's initial prognosis is left to emergency room physicians who provide only immediate emergency care. The door is open for big-time surprises. Many people thought to have serious brain damage recover better than anyone initially anticipated. Many who were thought to have just minor injuries don't ever recover fully.

That injured person in your life is much like a baby. Babies have obvious limitations and similarities to each other, but each has its own personality, distinct capabilities and hidden potential. Similarly, every survivor brings to the table a different history and a different set of circumstances leading up to and including the head trauma. And each will have his or her own path to recovery.

There is no comfortable way to watch someone you care about face a difficult recovery. Depending on the severity of the injury, many aspects of the survivor's life—as well as your own, and the relationship between the two of you—may undergo changes that will permeate many emotional levels.

There's a fine line between believing this is still the person you cared about before the injury and understanding that some of the rules now need to be changed. You may be seriously puzzled when you compare her actions and words now to her personality before the trauma. For example, I experienced bouts of surprising anger that were very unlike my mild temperament before the injury. I remember losing my temper one day over something quite insignificant, and my brothers thinking I was just in a bad mood or feeling grumpy. It wasn't that at all. They were simply playing by a set of rules that no longer applied.

The first priority is to assure the patient's safety and assess his ability to make competent and logical choices. You're likely to feel protective, maybe overly so. But, if he's capable of making appropriate decisions that don't put him in harm's way, he must be allowed that latitude. An adult patient especially needs to make some of his own choices and test his boundaries. Smothering and hiding him, even with the best of intentions, will only break his spirit and diminish his confidence.

You may have to make some changes around the patient's home. I had to have safety equipment installed in my bathroom. I moved my dishes down from the top shelves so I wouldn't have to reach up and lose my balance. I arranged furniture, cleared pathways, and installed handrails so I wouldn't stumble moving from room to room. I put night lights in the bathroom and bedroom to help me maneuver in the dark. I put phones in most of my rooms for easier access, especially in case of an emergency.

Most of my adjustments were made with my balance dysfunction in mind. So must decisions be made in each case that reflect the survivor's biggest challenges.

One of the greatest things you can do for the patient is simply to listen. Learn how she feels, encourage her to openly express what she is experiencing. Find out what frustrates her and what she has trouble with. Reinforce the idea that you are willing to assist her if she needs help with anything. Offer to attend appointments with her. Learn as much as you can and share with other members of the support group any information regarding head injury and the tendencies of its survivors. And, most importantly, try not to hold her up to comparison with her preaccident self. She's doing that already.

Your willingness to accept the injury is key. No matter how much you wish he had not been injured, you cannot change that. Through fear of the unknown, or unwavering hope, you will probably be inclined to promise him complete healing or prod him on to recover entirely. Be careful! One of the people in my cheering section kept telling me that I was "strong enough to beat this," that I had to "keep trying" and "work harder" in order to fully recover all I had lost. What was meant as encouragement and support made me feel as if I were failing to live up to expectations. There are things that will help, yes. But this isn't simply a matter of how many sit-ups you do or how many miles you run. In the end, some people will not heal entirely. Period.

Patients are bound to feel self-conscious as they begin to find limitations on how much they can do and what they have trouble with. It's important that they continue to be included in their social circles to the greatest possible extent. Head injury recovery is an *isolating* process. It seeks to dismantle the patient and everyone in his or her life. It is powerful and it is hungry.

Members of the help squad have the difficult challenge of nurturing the injury survivor's life, even as it changes because of the injury. The survivor might not be able to play in the traditional volleyball game at the traditional family picnic. Too many people and too much noise at the beach may overwhelm her. If the patient is having a difficult time visiting places that remind her of things she can no longer share, take the family somewhere new. Put off that picnic for a week or a month. Do it next summer! Some of the best plans are the ones that are never made.

Maybe this is the perfect time to explore places that are new to all of you; places that will forge new shared memories instead of resurrecting old ghosts.

It is often the case that when someone is ill, his obvious needs become priorities for everyone around him. Caregivers can end up sick or exhausted or burned out because they abandon their own lives and their own needs for the sake of the patient. I know I exhausted the people taking care of me because my needs were so great, and most everyone I knew lived 45 minutes away. Even though my bosses, Diana and Kris, had jobs, families and lives of their own, they were taking me to appointments and cooking my meals and taking care of my dogs and shopping for groceries and picking up medications.

It's important that the help be given, certainly. But it's more important that it be shared and changed and kept as fresh as possible. It helps no one to burn yourself out. You cannot be upbeat and supportive if you are feeling resentful that you have no time to yourself. The patient will end up feeling guilty and the environment will become tense. Nobody needs that. The situation is challenging enough as it is.

Some head injury survivors display behavior that is different from what you've known of them, even inappropriate, and it's difficult not to blame them or take their actions personally. Some patients become sexually provocative or explicit. Some who previously talked like preachers may suddenly break into torrents of swearing.

Doctors can identify the different regions of the brain and the specific behaviors each region influences. But it's mostly by trial and error that we figure out which environments or situations trigger aberrant behavior, and what remedies might help.

In my case, sudden fits of anger or weeping would overtake me. It was hard for my friends not to take it personally or wonder what the hell I was getting all bent out of shape about. I had them on eggshells. After a while they knew that when too many people were talking at the same time, when plans changed, if I was in a crowd or a foreign situation, or if something was happening that mildly annoyed *them*, I was probably enraged. With a little practice, we found that when I started tapping my cane, or got a certain look on my face, they needed to divert me to somewhere quiet and peaceful. Or they would bring me home, so I could regain my composure.

It took a while for them not to take it to heart when I grew angry with them or in their presence. And it was hard for me to watch myself carry on like that; at some level, even when the inner storm was at its peak, I knew damn well my behavior was excessive and inappropriate.

At the beginning of this chapter, I likened head injury survivors to newborns. By no means am I saying we're a bunch of babies. What I am saying is that parents have to allow their children to grow up, but they also have to monitor and provide some control over the process and events involved. There's a fine line to walk, and the goal is to neither overmanage nor undermanage. The relationship between caregiver and brain injury survivor is quite analogous, even though the ages may be different.

And eventually, as with a child, the strings of dependency must begin to be severed. I don't know the exact signpost that indicates it's time to start. It's a process, not a discrete event, and a slow process at that. It might take weeks …months …years. And it can be hard as hell to break the parental pattern and allow survivors to tackle the world without you battling to clear the brush in front of them.

But when the time's right, you gotta let 'em fly! Yes, they might take one step out of the nest and fall on their faces. But as long as they are willing to try, and are stubborn in their desire to pursue their own lives, they must be allowed to test those wings.

I have been called many things during my recovery. "Stubborn" is probably the most printable. I walked too far. I navigated across busy roads I had no business being on. I climbed up ladders and changed light bulbs. I tried to shovel snow and mow my hilly lawn. I went places and did things I was told not to do.

And often I failed. I have ended up face down in a culvert on the side of a road, covered in garbage. I've lain naked on my bathroom floor after a fall, hoping I wasn't hurt so that no one would have to find me lying naked on my bathroom floor.

Early on, friends would step in and refuse to allow me to do things they thought might be dangerous. I was so busy shrugging off the injury and denying its effects that, more than once, I could easily have gotten myself killed. But somewhere along the way, I found the elusive line between what I wanted to do and what I actually *could* do. I grudgingly accepted help for things I needed assistance with, and that was hard. I fought to do the things I could, and sometimes they weren't easy. And my friends released me, little by little.

I could have continued to allow them to do everything for me and, bless their hearts, they would have. But the time came when I had to take that step out of the nest. It didn't mean they stopped worrying. Or caring. It only meant we were making progress. And even though I did (often literally) fall on my face, their willingness to allow me to test my boundaries played a significant role in reestablishing my life.

Finally, caregivers, we brain injury survivors will probably never find a way to thank you for everything you do. But none of it gets overlooked. And to the extent our possibly impaired memories permit a promise like this to be carried out, none of it will ever be forgotten.

The New Year

THE CLUBHOUSE TURN

New Year's Day, 1997

I hesitate to start a new journal, as it serves to remind me that my travels continue. I didn't choose this road, and this year I must find the exit ramp. I don't believe in my heart of hearts that my balance retraining is going to help. That either means I am finally becoming realistic, or that I have lost hope. Either way, I will not depend on its success to define my own success.

New Year's Eve felt so welcome; perhaps a signal to an end. I'm terribly determined to get busy living. I must no longer feel victim to the impact of loss or the grief that proves so disabling. I may recognize their presence, but I can't succumb to them for days and weeks on end. They might nip at my heels, but I will beat them, chase them away. Be gone! Off with your heads!

I feel like the Red Wings did last year. They were supposed to win it all. They were shoo-ins. Everything was supposed to come together for them—and they lost. I, with my "mild" injury, was supposed to come together as well. I was supposed to recover wholly and did not. I could

131

probably talk for hours with Wings' captain Stevie Y. on how it feels to wonder, bewildered, how lofty expectations can breed such bitter disappointment.

1997 will be a year of answers to many of the questions '96 has posed: where I will live, what I will do for a living, how much more I will heal. I will continue to see Ginger, as she remains my link from past to future. We are challenged to find the right key for me to sing in. I tell myself we will.

The anniversary of my accident is just four weeks away. I don't know if I'll do anything ceremonial for it. I think the fact that it took six months to really comprehend the power of my injury and its impact makes the actual day less potent. That day I was actually thinking I had escaped almost unscathed ...

I haven't missed a Wings game since my accident. They have struggled, too, and I wonder if they, like me, can find in themselves a way to seize the underdog role and turn it on its ear. Sometimes just easing the expectations creates an environment for success. I think I started to improve the most when I accepted the fact that I might not. *Carpe diem!*

I found a verse that touched me and I sent framed prints of it to my friends for Christmas. It is my mantra for the New Year, for my new life ...

Live with intention,
Walk to the edge
Listen hard,
Practice wellness
Play with abandon,
Laugh
Choose with no regret,
Appreciate your friends
Do what you love,
Live as if this is all there is.

—Mary Anne Hershey

May 15, 1998

Lesson # 324: Don't get your oil changed late in the day when you know you should already be in bed.

I pulled up to Uncle Ed's Oil Change. It was on the way home and I was already caught in rush-hour traffic. I figured I could waste a little time off the road. Kill two birds with one stone.

So there I am and it wasn't two minutes into it that I knew I shouldn't have done this. The guy was all perky, pretending to accompany the obnoxiously loud music blasting in the garage with his clipboard guitar. He wanted the year of my car, my license plate number and how many miles since the last oil change. I read him the miles on my odometer instead and couldn't remember my license plate number to save my life. I got the year of the car right, thank God, and he left me alone.

I sat in the car, window up, trying to focus. I was sweating and panicking, trying to think of what he might ask me next. Men in oil-covered uniforms were darting in and out, attending to cars on either side of me. Out of nowhere the clipboard rock star reappeared at my window and motioned for me to roll it down. I turned the car all the way on and he gave me that, "You are a dumdum" look. He instructed me just to turn on the power, roll the window down, turn off the power, pop the hood—*Where is the hood latch?* Have to move the car up just a little, turn the key just to power and put it in neutral, what kind of oil did we use before, unlock the passenger's door so we can lubricate the hinges ...

He was now in slow motion. I was watching him talk, but only hearing "$8F6g@#$vhfy*&^n(N6tfg." I closed my eyes and cursed myself for thinking this would be a good idea. My head pounded and my ears were buzzing. Houston, we have a problem. I reclined my seat.

I woke up to the clipboard man pounding on my window, "Ma'am, Ma'am!!! Are you OK?" I was embarrassed and discombobulated. Two other attendants had now taken emergency positions at the front of my car. I looked at the rock star, my eyes glazed, and said something in Swahili. I managed to roll the window down and give him my money. He said something about a valve that needed to be replaced soon and I promised I would take care of that (when hell freezes over) right away, thank you for telling me.

He finally opened that garage sliding door, and I pulled out and onto a side street. I slept for almost two hours.

I ended up healing 100 percent. I won the lottery and I'm writing this book while sipping steaming glögg in front of a roaring fire at my lakefront log cabin in Sweden.

OK, OK, I'm kidding.

I would love to tell you I healed 100 percent. While this book was meant to describe my personal experience with brain injury, it was also meant to encourage and provide hope for injury survivors and the people who support them. It would have been a nice touch to be able to say I'm fully back to my preinjury self. But in many ways it's best that I'm not.

Truth is, the journey continues. There are good days and bad days. No, strike that. There are good and bad parts of each day. The other week I accidentally took the medicine my vet prescribed for my dog, Coda. The good news is I won't get hip dysplasia.

I still experience inappropriate anger. Dr. Cini has me taking Zoloft so I will play nicely with the other children. Diana suggested I bring what's left of my entertainment center to my new home so I'll have something to take my frustrations out on. Ginger suggested I get big pillows to beat up. All good ideas. Still, nothing could save my CDs last week. I got exercised about something, and they ended up flying like Frisbees out the back door and into the snow.

I continue to take medication for headaches. I still fall when I get too cocky and try to carry too much or go too fast. When I think I'm Wonder Woman again, I start three projects and end up finishing none and causing four more.

Every busy morning gives way to an afternoon of mental oatmeal. I pay for the times when I don't budget my productivity or calculate my itinerary closely enough. Before my appliances were delivered, I went to the laundromat. I was thinking I had an awful lot of laundry until I opened the first bag and found pizza boxes and newspapers in it. I'd brought along my garbage as well as my dirty clothes.

Every time I try to play by the old rules, I am reminded in some way that my injury has not healed completely and likely never will. I find reminders of challenges and failures everywhere. I've lost most of my china to ill-fated snits. I have two kitchen chairs left and my television teeters on the sad remains of what used to be my entertainment center. My body is constantly mending new and used bruises from falls. I still get tired and jumbled and frustrated.

I have trouble focusing my sense of orderliness on the right priorities. Before the accident, I knew I had to be highly meticulous and detail-oriented in my work. When I was off the job, I was pretty laid-back and casual. Now it seems I can't turn that switch on and off consistently and appropriately. I may organize the beverages in my refrigerator according to category, size and alphabet, then turn around and pay no attention to my checkbook. At this moment I am trying to find where I spent $1,150. I have no idea. It sure didn't go to bills!

A year ago I might have accepted my friends' proposal that they look over or handle my finances. Today I choose to do it myself. It's not lack of trust in them; it's having trust in me. It's accepting the possibility that I might fail because the prospect of succeeding is so captivating, so necessary, so delicious. I will find a way.

I'm making plans. I have expectations of myself again and I'm lengthening my strides. I feel more confident and competent. I don't interpret difficulties and failures as implying my lack of character (which doesn't mean I don't get *frustrated* by them). I'm better able to separate what I *won't* do from what I *can't* do, and what I shouldn't do with what I'd better. I'm able to laugh at myself again. (When I can't laugh at myself, I drive up to a valet, leave my car and watch the faces of the attendants as they realize there are gas pedals on each side of the brake. *Then* I laugh.)

I recently sold my home and moved closer to my family. I've lowered my mortgage payment since the next job is likely to pay considerably less than the last one.

The move itself represented many things. It was a financially sound decision and it afforded me some emotional closure. It feels like I've left an arena of listlessness, self-pity and anger behind, like I've chosen to move on and start life again. If the weight this took off me could be reflected in actual, physical pounds, I would be positively svelte.

Of course, the move presented its own challenges. By now my friends are old pros at knowing what help I require. They painted places I couldn't reach and carried boxes I had no business carrying. They installed the safety equipment, tightened loose handles and put in bright lighting.

Surviving those first few weeks surrounded by chaos was difficult. I've worked to entrench myself in routine and eliminate spontaneity, keeping things simple and predictable. The sight of stacked boxes and the unfamiliarity of new rooms sent me into dithers. I continue to remind myself that I've come through worse.

I am currently in therapy at the Spectrum Rehabilitation Center in Southfield, Michigan. My course of treatment is designed to assist me in my pursuit of a new career. I still can't juggle so I suppose the circus is out. I don't imagine the Wings would consider a 32-year-old towel woman. This is when I wish I'd listened to Aunt Helen and learned to play the accordion.

These next few months will be a sifting process of sorts: strengths, challenges, likes, dislikes. I'm struggling to find a consistent level of productivity. I seem to be at my most efficient between three and six in the morning. Maybe I could deliver the Detroit Free Press.

If no company will dare employ me because I remain an insurance risk (for falling), I will consider starting my own home-based business or determine the need to use a wheelchair while at work (did I really say that?). And no matter what else, I'll write.

I'm now close enough to cook occasional meals and do a few loads of laundry for my dad. I'm grateful for the opportunity to give something back after all my parents did for me—another example of some good that came out of all this.

After 18 months I got my driver's license back. My retraining was completed through a program at Providence Hospital. I had three instructors: Mark, Margaret and Lesley. They were so amazingly calm and patient that I thought Dr. Cini must have had them on Zoloft as well.

Margaret determined that I would need to utilize a left-foot accelerator because my right foot didn't respond appropriately to the tests she administered. Mark started me off in an empty parking lot. The first couple of days he kept asking, "Kara, why do you keep pressing both the gas and brake pedals at the same time?" It was weird enough being in a car again, let alone trying to learn a new way to drive it.

Lesley supervised my on-road training. We spent several weeks on sparsely traveled side streets, practicing parking, using turn signals, getting acclimated again to traffic. I graduated to main roads and eventually the freeway. After passing the road test, I was able to reapply for a Michigan driver's license. I was required to take another road test, as well as a written one. I was so excited that I studied the driver's handbook as if it were a bar exam.

I have a wheelchair on my license plate but I try not to park in the first spot unless there is ice and snow. I can even drive through the intersection where my accident took place without wincing and singing "Amazing Grace" (well, most of the time anyway).

The first few times back on the road felt so foreign—almost like I was a criminal, sneaking back on the road when everyone was looking for me in the ditches. There is a rhythm to driving that I had lost. Like a 16-year-old kid, I had to think about everything, where once it had all been second nature.

I was very fortunate not to experience the paralyzing fear that commonly grips drivers after a serious auto accident. There was one woman who spent the first six months of her retraining just getting comfortable walking up to the vehicle. I really felt sympathy for her. But I had a bogeyman of my own to deal with. As exciting as it was to anticipate reclaiming my independence, I had to shoo away that ugly little monster telling me I was out there again. On the road. One intersection from disaster.

I was never much of a drinker (my friends might laugh when they read that). I haven't even had a beer since my accident and I doubt I'll ever drink alcoholic beverages again. A "cold one" wouldn't be a wise chaser for all the medication I take. And balance is hard enough as it is. If a police officer ever asked me to walk a straight line or sing the alphabet when I'm tired and talking Swahili, I'd be hard-pressed to explain myself.

I haven't lost all that weight I put on. I now have three sets of clothes: preaccident, early recovery and waterproof pup tent. I'm working on it. Somebody once said, "If God had wanted us to touch our toes, He'd have put them on our knees!" Works for me.

Since you're reading this, I have witnessed the publication of my first book. My body is probably more like *Moby Dick* than the book is, but I am delighted nonetheless. Writing it was a lot more difficult than I imagined and a lot more satisfying. I didn't know what to expect of it. At various stages the process was disappointing, painful, rewarding. Therapeutic for sure. The fact that I dreamed of writing before the accident, then realized that dream after it, means the world to me.

I spent this past spring watching my beloved Red Wings pummel Colorado and sweep the Philadelphia Flyers to capture the Stanley Cup championship (more about this in the Epilogue). We waited 42 years to bring Lord Stanley back to Detroit. Watching our Captain, Steve Yzerman, hoist that Cup and skate around the rink was truly inspiring. I could relate to the relief in his expression: *the demons have been dispatched.* It's nice to think that neither one of us will dread waking up each morning to questions we have no answers for. He silenced his critics by adding the Cup to his Hall of Fame résumé. I am silencing mine by giving myself a break here and there and realizing I am, by far, my worst critic. Maybe I'm coming to peace with everything. Then again, maybe it's just the Zoloft kicking in.

Sometimes I still find it hard to believe how much time has passed since the day I was hurt. I have found that my injury is as much about the car accident as a marriage is about the wedding day. It's simply the first page in a new chapter.

During the first months, while I wondered why Fate decreed my injury, I came up with usable temporary rationalizations. Then my mom passed away and I immediately knew what larger purpose all this served.

Had I not been injured, work would have continued to consume my time—holidays and weekends, mornings and nights. I would have continued to live far enough away from family to make visits infrequent. And when we got together, conversations would have remained in the safe, shallow waters of everyday life. We would have continued to muse about the weather, the latest game or movie, or hot political scandal.

Instead I lost my health, my career and my home. I lost the abilities that had served me so well. I found myself back home, within five minutes of where I grew up. Doctors had run out of therapies to try, tests to administer, and hope to give that I would be who I was three years ago. I settled into the medications that controlled the symptoms that refused to heal. I settled into the routines that kept me safe. I settled into the circle of people who accepted and adjusted to the new me. And my mom and I were able to spend precious time together.

The visits I shared with Mom the last six months before her death, the smiles we traded, were priceless. How ironic that when neither of us could speak clearly and correctly, we said the most important words of our lives to each other. We ended a lingering suffering. She found her peace and I found mine. And largely because of that, I no longer ask, "Why?" Instead I say, "Thank you."

I wanted to end with something special; something poignant, a sentence or two that would just make people's lights go on. I wanted to wrap up with a great, romantic finish, the kind that leaves you delighted you read the book and sad that it had to end.

But I looked inside and found little closure. That's the tragedy of brain injury. It doesn't tie up neatly in ribbons and bows. It's the guest that stays long beyond its welcome. It's the scratchy throat that lingers all winter and into spring.

So no boffo ending, but let me close with two important messages. First, to all brain injury survivors: you are part of an enormous community. There are professionals in every capacity who can help you through this. And you have the company and understanding of those of us who sit quietly next to you on the bus. Our ultimate wish, our ultimate vision, is that no one ever has to face recovery from a brain injury. For now, the wish and the vision are simply that no one has to face it alone.

And second, to everyone else: never forget that life doesn't follow the plans we make just because we make them. We have to allow for change, prepare for it, seek positive results from it. We have to understand that tragedy, sadness and unexpected challenge may wreak havoc at any time, and leave us facing hard work to recover a life.

That morning I didn't imagine that the person I was would be gone forever, so I made no preparations. I hadn't saved enough money; I hadn't planned for my retirement; I didn't know enough about my insurance policies; I didn't call my friends and family to tell them I love them; I had no will; I hadn't cleaned my house. I thought I had all the time in the world when pretty much all I had going for me was a seat belt and Someone keeping an eye out for me. It makes petty fights and silly grudges and those times we leave the house without a goodbye kiss worth reconsidering.

We don't know what tomorrow will bring. We have no idea how many near misses we've already escaped, or what waits around the corner, whispering our name in the darkness. We can become paranoid, I suppose. We can stay in our homes and refuse to be injured, refuse to be changed, refuse to be damaged. Or we can *live*, even if unexpected circumstances throw us sinking curve balls. We can be smart and stop thinking we're untouchable. We can do the little things that eliminate many of the needless accidents we read about every day in the newspaper. And we can surround ourselves with quality people who will help us, and whom we will help, should Fate put either of us aboard the bus at its next stop.

As for me, this verse by Fran Sloan says it all:

> Come to the edge,
> Life said.
> They said,
> We are afraid.
> Come to the edge,
> Life said.
> They came.
> It pushed them ...
> And they flew.

Epilogue

LORD, PLEASE MEND OUR BROKEN WINGS

I have lived in Michigan all my life. I remember walking into Tiger Stadium as a kid and seeing the outfield grass for the first time—the bright powdered chalk lines, the manicured infield, the stadium lights. They took my breath away. Still do.

I remember my parents buying me one of those miniature bats with Al Kaline's signature on it. I was barely able to see over the guardrail, eating hot dogs steamed in foil wrappers. I'd wear my Detroit Tigers cap with the Olde English "D," my name printed neatly under the perfectly creased bill. I'd watch beach balls come floating out of the bleachers, and listen to the crack of the bat, the hum of the crowd, the singsong peddlers irresistibly chanting, "Hot dog, getcher hot dog here …"

I grew up eating Mom's chili and watching University of Michigan football on autumn Saturdays. The leaves would turn brilliant reds and golds, crisply crunching underfoot. Mom would yell, "Go get 'em, boys!" and we'd laugh at Bo stomping up and down the sidelines arguing a call.

I celebrated our baseball World Champion Tigers in '84, and a few years later, the back-to-back NBA basketball titles of the "Bad Boys" Pistons.

Knocking off Notre Dame (or trying to) early in the season and charging late to beat Ohio State for the Big Ten Title are still year-after-year highlights. A New Year's Day trip to Pasadena for the Wolverines always outranks any New Year's Eve plans. And watching the Lions' annual Thanksgiving Day game is a sacred tradition.

Detroit is a passionate, knowledgeable sports town. We take deep pride in the rich traditions associated with our teams. Our city has provided some of the finest athletes in professional sports history.

Like most sports fans, if I'm lucky enough to get within 10 feet of one of our stars, I get all goofy and pie-eyed. There is something about celebrity that makes us all feel 12 again. And when you have such consummate professionals as Alan Trammell, Barry Sanders, Joe Dumars and Steve Yzerman, you enjoy their special presence. It is exhilarating.

But even among all the great teams of our past, the 1997 Detroit Red Wings may have captured local hearts like no other—in my lifetime, anyway. Our quest for the Stanley Cup brought the city *together.* The vibes were powerful, shared, unprecedented. Parts of Michigan, especially Detroit, have an intensely unfavorable reputation: drug-infested, gang-inhabited, war zone-dangerous, desperate, explosive. To see people embrace each other and discard their racial, economic and cultural differences for two months during one glorious spring was magnificent, a rare and unforgettable magic. Those who experienced it will never tire of retelling the story.

During that season I often felt the Wings mirrored my own hopes and battles. I didn't care that it sounded silly. I watched every game they played and it was almost a welcome coincidence that they seemed to struggle when I did. When they would go four or five games without a loss, I frequently seemed to be rallying with my own "winning streaks." Admittedly, it was a little weird. Admittedly, I didn't care.

When their run in the 1997 Stanley Cup playoffs began, they represented the goals that I, too, was chasing: dismissal of past failure and the rebirth of hope. We both had momentum now. They battled and overcame pain, disappointment, struggle and doubt—the same enemies I fought to defeat. They made me feel wonderfully alive, part of a city witnessing something truly special. Making history. Together we would raise the roof of expectation.

When the Wings swept the Philadelphia Flyers in the '97 finals, I shared that moment with my friends. We hugged and cried, celebrating and hearing honking horns long into the night. We had come to love these guys in red and white sweaters almost like brothers. They were unique in that they refused to buy into their celebrity. Their appreciation of our support felt genuine. Our affection felt reciprocated. They were humble and polite and so refreshingly different from the greedy, self-absorbed stars who so densely populate professional sports today. Mickey Redmond, our long-time announcer and former Red Wing great, may have said it best when he called the relationship between this team and its fans "personal."

Like the knee-high kids who wait in the tunnel of Joe Louis Arena hoping for their heroes to walk by, I, too, wanted to be close to them. To sip from the Cup they invited us to share. To feel the camaraderie and focus and drive that creates champions. But while I wished many times that I might one day meet them, never in my wildest nightmare did I think I would find myself sitting next to any of them on the bus.

As the deliriously happy state continued to celebrate its Stanley Cup championship, our victorious heroes met for one last dinner party before going their separate ways for the summer. During the off season, each would be allowed to host the Cup for a day. Some would share it with family and friends. Some would sleep with it. Some would take it to hospitals where sick kids in need of inspiration would get to take a picture with it. Our Russian players planned to pool their days and take Lord Stanley to their homeland for the first time in history. Local news stations planned to cover the Cup's maiden voyage to Russia and broadcast an event filled with marvelous "one world" symbolism: the Stanley Cup in Red Square. The stage was set for the best summer of those players' lives.

At that last party they did the right thing. To ensure road safety for all and avoid "driving while intoxicated" risks, knowing there would be no shortage of celebratory drinks and toasts, a transportation company was hired to drive them home after their dinner. But sometimes doing the right thing just isn't enough. Tragedy struck anyway. The limousine carrying defensemen Vladimir Konstantinov and Slava Fetisov, and team masseur Sergei Mnatsakanov, veered off the road. It hit a tree while traveling over 50 miles an hour.

News of the accident broke into our homes like ruthless burglars, quickly stealing the joy from our hearts and rendering our precious silver worthless. Fetisov's injuries proved relatively minor, but Konstantinov and Mnatsakanov suffered life-threatening closed head injuries. We watched, desperately searching for information and fielding calls long into the night. A family emergency had erupted: our brothers were hurt.

Local news stations headed straight to the hospital. Footage of Red Wings' owner Mike Ilitch and members of the team rushing to Beaumont Hospital seared our minds and sickened our stomachs with the same intensity with which the week of celebration had wrapped our hearts in red and white jubilation. Hundreds of shocked fans, not knowing what to do, were drawn to the accident site with candles and souvenirs that, only hours before, had delighted. Some stood silently in the hospital parking lot. Strangers hugged, prayed and cried together. They came to share, to console, to be consoled. That's what happens when someone in the family gets hurt.

That first mention of head injury took my breath away and left me sitting on the couch in stunned silence. Flashbacks of my own accident flooded over me. Many of my friends told me later they thought of me right away when they heard the news. I knew instinctively that hundreds of thousands of brain injury survivors would soon be making room on the bus for two of our heroes. "Damn you, injury! Damn you!" I cried.

We had waited 42 years to bring the Stanley Cup home to Detroit. Now that same loyalty, patience, hope and determination would have to be called upon again. It felt so sadly ironic.

People easily understand the kind of bruises and cuts that Vladdie inflicted and received with his powerful checks into the boards. (His nickname is "the Vladiator.") And many of us have suffered the types of injuries that Sergei helped heal in the team's training room. But, like my own family and friends almost two years before, most of the team's followers had no understanding of the significance of those initial reports. Closed head injury? What does that mean?

That first night, a reporter asked if Vladdie would play hockey again in the fall. I was enraged—not by his lack of understanding, but by his wrongly ordered priorities.

Much has been written about the adventuresome paths that took five of our Wings from Russia's famous Red Army teams and the Soviet National World Champion squads to the National Hockey League. We have told grand tales of how their journeys have afforded them the fortunes of our generous culture. We are proud that they are able to send hope and help back home, in the form of hockey equipment and money, to thousands of kids who would otherwise have no chance to follow in their footsteps.

I knew that Vladimir and Sergei would now reap the most precious of the benefits they had secured with their talents: top medical care in their moment of need. Before the ambulances had even reached the hospital, our state's most noted neurological specialists were consulting on the course of their treatment. From the beginning, we were assured that the very best of care and expertise would be on the bench behind them.

But my own experience told me that much of their recovery would not come from the skills of prominent medical professionals. More in their favor, perhaps, would be the overwhelming embrace of their friends and "extended family," now numbering in the millions. As they inched toward recovery, their support system would need to reactivate the patience, loyalty and hopeful determination it had bestowed on the long-suffering team.

The accident happened less than a week after we won the Stanley Cup. We were filled with surprise at how something we thought meant everything for 42 years now meant so little, really. And we learned that our care and concern for these players and their families extended far beyond what they did in their uniforms. Our prayers and thoughts were and are not just for defensemen and trainers. They are for men. Young, strong men with jobs and families, hopes and dreams, and dreams that finally came true. They are for people who become, in one awful moment, just like anyone else caught in random, senseless tragedy and directed to a seat on the bus.

As coverage in Detroit faded from hourly updates to frustrating reports on the lack of obvious progress, we began to realize that recovery for these two would not mean looking forward to training camp, regular-season travel and another run at Lord Stanley. Detroit was beginning to understand that while they might eventually recover, a realistic notion of "recovery" might require us to change the working definition of that word.

While many viewers puzzled that first night, everyone in the brain injury community—survivors and their families, medical, legal and mental health professionals—all felt the painful bite of those initial news reports. Knowing something of what lay ahead did not comfort in that moment; it sadly confounded. From the moment the limousine crashed, every morning began and every evening ended with updates and reports on how our guys were recovering and what a head injury actually is. Information on brain injury was everywhere: television, radio, newspapers, in the minds and on the lips of an entire state. Our relatively obscure malady was suddenly front and center, but at a wrenching cost.

As I watched many of my own experiences play out on a large screen, I saw some of the same wonderful support dynamics reach out to embrace these new passengers on the bus. Anyone familiar with hockey will tell you of the animosity between the Colorado Avalanche and the Detroit Red Wings. It has stewed and boiled and bubbled over into moblike brawls and violent scrums. They have become bitter rivals, providing fans with classic hockey, heroic performances and bloody fisticuffs.

Yet when news of the Red Wings' accident spread, everyone in the NHL, including the Avalanche, quickly embraced the injured players in their fight to survive. At the 1997 National Hockey League Awards program, practically every award recipient paid tribute and offered prayers to our heroes and their families. These decorated, larger-than-life men, used to dueling on the ice like savage warriors, now wept with us. And Colorado, who on the ice would return every vicious hit the Vladiator laid out, sent a five-foot-high card signed by everyone in the organization and some of their fans, wishing a full recovery.

That is more than just class. It shows understanding that tragedy affects lives without regard to status, title, age, fortune—or the team jersey one is wearing.

Eventually we adjusted to the idea that our autumn banner-raising ceremony would lack some of the luster we had anticipated. It was now clear that Vladdie and Sergei faced a new and more fundamental set of challenges and priorities. Sadly, we acknowledged that reclaiming their familiar roles on our team was no longer a realistic goal.

Here in Detroit, a family of millions still consumes every morsel of information about Sergei and Vladdie. Months later, trees are still tied with big red bows. Newspapers continue to educate on brain trauma. People are quick to trade infrequent updates at dinner tables and water coolers. Signs in shops, picture windows and cars continue to send get-well wishes. Celebrities host events to help fund brain injury associations. We keep them in our minds, in our prayers, in the best of memories and the most determined of hopes.

❧

The Detroit Red Wings won their second consecutive Stanley Cup championship in 1998. All season long, behind their mighty winged sweaters beat hearts sickened by the loss of two members of their hockey family. Vladimir Konstantinov and Sergei Mnatsakanov were the silent voices of inspiration behind a team determined to give them another shot at the celebration cut short a year before by their devastating injuries.

Game Four of the finals was in Washington against the chippy Capitals. We were up three games to none and a sweep now seemed imminent, but a touch bittersweet. I think we all wanted the team to come back and win the Cup on home ice, although we knew the danger of tempting Fate and letting an opponent back in the series.

During the last period of that last game, faces started to look up from the ice toward an upper section of the seats. Slowly, as recognition swept through the arena, Vladimir Konstantinov, making his first game appearance since his injury, was helped up from his wheelchair: jersey number 16, standing in section number 16. There, amidst thousands of fans, our team was no longer on foreign ice, battling the home crowd of Washington. The players on both teams started rapping their sticks on the ice—their sign of recognition and respect. The crowd stood cheering, and the tears and the chills reached all the way back to Detroit.

As the final seconds ticked off the clock, our team rushed onto the ice, tossing gloves and sticks in the air. We were NHL champions again, and what came next epitomizes everything I have wanted to convey in this book.

Team captain Steve Yzerman graciously accepted the Stanley Cup trophy on behalf of the Detroit Red Wings. He raised it high above his head, circling the ice as flashes from thousands of cameras glinted off its gleaming silver. And then he turned and gave that Cup to Vladimir Konstantinov, who had been wheeled onto the ice to celebrate this moment with his teammates.

When I saw Vladdie with that Cup, I felt so deeply proud and moved. What an inspiration, what a joy, for those of us who work every day to recover our lives after brain injury. Here was this man, poised victoriously between who he had been and who he will be. Here was this man, still meaning so much to the people around him, still contributing to his team and to hockey fans everywhere.

Thousands of hands clapped while he sat in a wheelchair, just as they had when he flew around the boards in hockey skates. His teammates on the ice joined fans sitting in front of television sets from Washington to Detroit to Russia, wiping tears from their eyes.

In that moment, Vladdie symbolically did what all of us with that injury must do: find a way to connect preinjury and postinjury selves into a new, whole person, ready to carry on life. And that whole person, that wonderful entirety of experiences, held the Stanley Cup in his hands.

At the pep rally honoring the team after they won the '98 Stanley Cup, Detroit Red Wings' Associate Coach Dave Lewis read a poem he had written that captures Vladdie's spirit and reflects the wonderful treasures within all of us. The poem is about the challenge of achieving a championship, but I found in his words much about life and recovery. He responded warmly to my request to include his poem in this book. I hope it will touch you with the same power and strength that touched me. (The team's slogan for the season was Vladdie's number and "Believe." The title also refers to the 16 playoff game victories required to win the Stanley Cup.)

Believe in 16

Life is measured in time lines.
The birth of a child, the death of a loved one,
The day you were drafted.
Your first car, the day you were married.
The age that passes by 20, 30, 40 years.
Time never stops, it never will.
The time spent in June of 1997 will never be erased
From the memory of those who were there.
The hearts of so many beat as one.
Living each other's dream for more than 8 weeks.
The time was right, we made it right.
Sixteen victories in the Spring of '97
Look back ..it seems like yesterday.
Was it easy? No.
Was it rewarding? Yes.
So many emotions ran through that June.
Only you know what you left back at that time.
It starts again where it ended.
JLA, Joe Louis Arena.
Some have gone, others have arrived.
Time and changes seem to have something in common.
The new are excited for a chance.
The old are excited for the same chance.
This time, the vision may be clearer
But the route will be different.
It will be as challenging.
There are no shortcuts on this journey.
You will be tested and tested again.

You are the champions!
There are 15 other teams, 360 players,
That want their time in June.
16 victories, 16.
If we could stop time, we would, that June day.
Believe me when I say,
That we have two extra hearts to add to our roster.
Their names aren't listed.
The number has great significance.
They will always be there.
Life is measured in time lines.
Don't let this time slip away.

—*Dave Lewis*

Team Kara

MY BOOKENDS

I was putting together the office in my new home and realized I had no bookends. My computer is set up near the back of the house. Every time the dogs would run by to get out the back door, their tails would knock the bookcase and all my books would slide right off the edge and onto the floor.

Funny things, bookends. Those overlooked pillars of strength that unassumingly stand guard over our stored knowledge. We don't give them credit or even notice them until the dogs run by and everything hits the floor.

What began as a rather lengthy thank-you letter to my family and friends grew into a series of therapeutic homework assignments that helped me process my feelings during my recovery—and ultimately emerged as this book. It's fitting that while I've attempted to share what I've learned and give back a measure of what I've been given, standing lookout around me are my pillars of strength. My sentinels. My bookends. TEAM KARA.

Everything I've recounted in these chapters is encompassed and protected by these people, the sentries of my recovery. Their words, expertise, caring and humor have warmed and protected me as their words now surround mine. Knowing they would be there writing "front matter" and "back matter" (as my publisher, a rather technical fellow, calls it) made my voice clearer. Knowing they would be there in my life made my recovery that much more successful.

I asked some of the key TEAM KARA members to write contributions for this book, and here they are. Thanks, team, especially for the great second half.

Team Kara

NOTES FROM A PHYSICIAN

Every year, hundreds of thousands of people are diagnosed with closed head injuries. Many more go undiagnosed. And the frequency of this injury is rising. Growing awareness of shaken baby syndrome, sports-related head trauma, and the increased incidence of motor vehicle accidents have brought to light an injury that has long been shrouded in silence and misunderstanding.

Because closed head brain damage often reveals few, if any, visible signs of injury, survivors and those around them—family, friends and co-workers—may doubt the validity of the injury. This increases the risk that survivors will not receive proper treatment and adds to the devastating life disruption that head trauma delivers. Often the survivor must relearn the easiest tasks and devise new strategies to execute daily responsibilities.

Doubt and misunderstanding complicate the recovery, making it even more difficult for the survivor to accept, address and attack the challenges. When doubts and misunderstandings come from close family and friends, a crushing burden is added to the recovery process. *I'll Carry the Fork!* provides a much-needed resource, helping to dispel doubt and convert harmful *mis*-understanding to constructive understanding.

My sincerest thanks to Kara for having shared her pain and for being the teacher that she has become to all of us on TEAM KARA. Most of all, I would like to thank her for allowing me to participate in her care and recovery, and to be an important part of her life. She has shown us that great courage and strength can overcome even the most difficult challenges, especially when mixed with humor and helped along by supportive people. Kara's book is an inspiration to us all to not give up hope during our most troubling times.

—Sharon L. Cini, MD

Team Kara

Having worked in brain injury rehabilitation for the past 10 years at the Lakeland Center in Southfield, Michigan, I have assisted many patients and their families through the challenges, struggles, disappointments and triumphs of their recovery. Every patient and every family is deeply affected by the catastrophic event of a closed head injury.

Kara Swanson places this life-altering disaster in a new perspective. She grapples with her own issues and problems, and shares with her readers the day-to-day obstacles she works so tirelessly to overcome. Despite her failures and frustrations, she writes humorously—almost joyfully—about how she had to persevere to accomplish even the simplest of tasks, and gives us all hope that there *is* life after brain injury.

She lets us see, from the inside out, how life as she knows it is inexorably changed, and how she has adapted her own habits and behaviors to compensate for the faculties and abilities she has lost. She works daily to recover the "Kara of yesteryear," a job that will never be done. Given her conviction, strength and commitment to be the very best she can,

Kara imparts a message of encouragement and hope to all who have suffered this devastating injury—and to those families and friends who have worked through its consequences along with them.

Even those of you whose lives have not been touched by injury: *read this book!* You will be enriched and inspired by her persistent quest for "normalcy." And you will thank your lucky stars that your life has been spared the impact of such an event.

Celebrate Kara's remarkable achievements with her. You will laugh out loud as you learn how she creatively fumbles through the daily activities we all take for granted. You will cry in empathy as you admire her never-ending courage and determination. And you will find yourself cheering for her along with the rest of us on TEAM KARA.

—Adrienne Shepperd, RN, BSN, MSA
Director of Marketing
The Lakeland Center, Southfield, Michigan

Team Kara

NOTES FROM A CLINICAL PSYCHOLOGIST

Before her accident, Kara approached therapy with the determination of the A student and varsity athlete that she was. She was committed and punctual. She completed her homework between sessions. She even brought in great cups of coffee and chocolates.

We had always enjoyed a positive working relationship. I knew what my job was. I understood the goals of our work together. I was confident of my ability to help her use her writing skills to process the traumas in her past. I felt she was making progress in determining what she truly wanted to do in her lifetime. And I thought she was taking steps toward recognizing those "red lights" that had led her to our work together. But I wasn't prepared for the red light that came next.

When Kara returned to therapy after the accident, she had bruises on her face and arms, and was unsteady on her feet. She held her head to one side. She couldn't track our conversations and failed to mention that her physician, Dr. Cini, had diagnosed her as suffering from a closed head injury. I expected that in time she would return to her old self.

As the weeks went by, the clear-thinking, extremely focused client I had come to know did not re-emerge. However, many of the changes were subtle and she did her best to conceal them from me. She was still funny and articulate, though at times she struggled to find words. She tired easily and tended only to use about 20 minutes of each session productively. She would obsess about the details of my office: a crooked picture, a water stain on the wall, light switches. Her letters to me no longer revealed her emotional states but offered amusing suggestions for my office staff or commentaries on the cabbies who brought her to therapy.

She was anxious to drive again and return to her work and normal life. At first I believed she would be able to accomplish these things quickly. When she told me about the closed head injury and the potential for an extended leave of absence, I had only a vague idea of what to expect. I struggled to develop a new treatment plan.

There were other changes, too. Kara was more dependent, more guarded. She worked harder at presenting herself in a positive light and revealed fewer of her vulnerabilities.

Together we waited for the tests and therapies to reveal the full extent of the injury—what was probably permanent and what might be expected to heal. I found the uncertainty extremely frustrating and wanted to get on to the next stage of treatment. I can only imagine how frustrating the waiting and uncertainty is for survivors and their families. When the test results and prognosis came in, we recognized that Kara would not be returning to the job or the life she had known, and that the two of us would not be returning to the relationship structure we had known either.

What made the psychotherapy different was that much of what she was experiencing was organically driven. I needed help. I sought advice and supervision. I talked to colleagues who worked exclusively with individuals with brain trauma. I was beginning to think Kara might benefit more by working with someone with more expertise. I was confident in the work we had done since the accident, but I didn't know where to go next.

I was focused on helping her process her feelings of helplessness and anger, and providing support during this very difficult time. But now she needed to get on with the process of learning to live with her injury. She would need to employ behavioral strategies to cope with her deficits. I have little background or interest in behavioral psychology, so I questioned my ability to make any meaningful contribution. I wasn't even sure what I *didn't* know or what questions to ask.

What was Kara doing while I was questioning my role? She didn't understand the diagnosis any more than I did. Initially, she refused to accept that her brain had been injured. Then she began looking for her own answers. She relentlessly quizzed her treating physicians. She went to medical libraries and read about brain injuries. She was *waiting,* going through tests and treatments and *waiting* for approvals for more tests and *waiting* for answers and *waiting* for more approvals, more tests and more treatments. The waiting seemed at times interminable. When no other help was forthcoming, she tried to devise her own treatment.

Early on, I couldn't tell which symptoms were reactions to the losses she was experiencing and which were organically based. I needed to learn when to recommend medical consultation; when to step in and help her develop and reinforce the use of new coping mechanisms; when to help her set goals; when to encourage movement toward them; when to *back off;* and when to just listen.

I believe that as both a therapist and a person, the greatest asset I can bring to any relationship is curiosity, a desire to understand. At times the most important thing I could do for Kara was just be genuinely interested in what this was like for her. Other days I merely provided a place where she didn't have to be grateful and strong.

I had read that irrational mood swings and rage were to be expected and were difficult to manage. This sounded unlikely for Kara, who had typically approached enraging situations with steely silence. In the weeks before the accident, she had filed a formal complaint for some women on her staff who were experiencing sexual harassment. That was Kara angry: organized, composed and calculating. However, new and unpredictable patterns began to emerge that we would have to understand and that she would need to learn to manage.

We read that staying motivated was frequently a problem after brain injury. I had seen clients lose focus and motivation when depression became chronic, or when they were given long-term medical leave. At first, Kara was anxious to get back to her life. But as more data became available about her injury, it became clear that Kara was not destined to be able to return to her job or the life she had known.

My job now was to help her accept the cognitive, emotional, physical and interpersonal consequences of her injury, and develop strategies to cope with her new limits. It was a long time and a lot of *waiting* before anyone would say what those limits might be. I was concerned about the concept of accepting limits, but equally concerned that Kara find a way to deal with the frustrations. It became clear she would never regain all of her previous functioning. She would need to find ways to celebrate small steps as progress.

Well-meaning family and friends who said they knew she could beat this thing made her feel overwhelmed, inadequate, misunderstood and alone. She was also devastated by the losses: participating in sports (her great passion), her career, her home, a solid income, the prospect of a new job, her mobility—her independence. All the markers of her achievements were gone.

She could no longer screen out background noise. She was distractible, with very limited endurance. The bouts of rage we had been warned about were becoming alarmingly familiar. She couldn't do more than one thing at a time. This for a woman who had previously planned and managed large catering operations, with a staff of hundreds, and worked countless 80-hour weeks.

Many individuals have been able to overcome seemingly insurmountable odds by refusing to accept the limits of their diagnosis. Knowing Kara and her determination, I thought she was just that kind of individual. The challenge—and the paradox—was how to help Kara accept limitations, yet not be defined by them.

However, one set of limitations was essential: she had to learn to recognize danger and respond appropriately. Kara was ignoring her balance problems, climbing on chairs to change light bulbs, or trying to climb through a window to help her father when his garage door failed to open. Red lights were figuratively blinking everywhere and she paid them little heed. This sounded like the Kara I had known so well. In her attempt not to be victimized, to seem unaffected by the accident, she was putting herself in very precarious situations. Another paradox: while it was exasperating to see her repeat old patterns we thought were changing prior to her injury, I took some comfort in recognizing parts of Kara that remained the same.

My supervisor's voice rang in my ear: "We only have one or two issues that we keep playing out over and over during our lifetime." Kara was fighting to maintain her independence, but everyday household tasks were now a hazard. My job was to help her recognize a whole new set of red lights. I had to guide her along the fine line between coping with a changed reality while not letting it completely control her life. She had to find a new path; the old one had come to a dead end.

It took a year after the accident before she began to accept that her future would be radically different from her past. She began to work with an alternative vocational therapist, someone to guide her back into the work force. His role was to help her identify and define what was professionally possible. Mine was to help her deal with emotional barriers.

There was a conflict between the two objectives. Emotionally, she wanted to *write*. But understandably, the vocational therapist encouraged her to pursue something more practical, perhaps using her catering management skills. Also, due to her balance problems, the other members of the treatment team insisted Kara use a wheelchair—at least in the workplace. She refused.

I encouraged her to be realistic about danger and adapt accordingly. I gently asked if she might be ignoring those red lights again. She became scared and angry. Early in her hospital and rehabilitation therapies, she would come into my office and describe how she was convinced she would end up "putting pens together" or be pushed into a life of a therapist's choosing, not hers. Initially, no one wanted her to put much hope in becoming a writer; it wasn't practical or dependable. People felt she needed a regular job with a reliable income.

Kara has a history of doing what is expected of her and not always following her own counsel. She was afraid that if she took her vocational therapist's initial recommendations, she would abandon her own dreams.

But Kara also has a feisty, oppositional streak. I wanted to mobilize and ignite this part of her. I challenged her to make her counselors eat their words. But I was cautious, too, afraid for her financial stability. I knew that the insurance settlement would provide only a meager income, and that her checks were frequently delayed for months. Being aware of her writing ambitions and talent, I talked with her about her novel and ideas for other literary efforts, but also about jobs for writers that might be more dependable, such as journalism. She was frustrated with me, now, too. I wasn't getting it! One day I received this letter:

> Dear Ginger,
>
> I have given everyone the impression that my only real reason for not wanting to go back to work in catering or any regular job is because of the wheelchair.
>
> That is only a part of it. Truthfully I am scared.
>
> I don't want to fail.
>
> I fear being with a bunch of people in a busy workplace (like when you mentioned a newspaper) and becoming overwhelmed. The noise, commotion … I get frustrated and panicky and angry. I hate the noise. I hate the buzz.
>
> I see myself calling in sick on the mornings when my headache won't go away, or when I can't feel my feet and won't drive.
>
> I fear a boss reprimanding my failure to remember something, or my need for him/her to talk more slowly or go over directions more than once.

I fear being with people who don't know I was once good. Who will see the things I am not good at. I fear having work be the only thing I do, when one drive or one project now sends me to bed for four hours.

I've never been one to call in sick or need someone to look over my shoulder. I have never been unpredictable or unreliable and I have lost my confidence.

And so, in the spirit of Spectrum [Rehabilitation Center], I look for ideas that will build on my *strengths.* Please help me to not waste this time and my life any further, Ginger. Please help me not to fuck up this opportunity. Help me to find some good in this experience and use it to really accomplish something.

Thanks,

Kara

After reading this letter, I knew she needed to take a risk to regain some of her confidence. The *right* risk would help her feel excited and alive again. I urged her to listen to her own voice. And after reading her manuscript, her vocational counselor swung into full support behind her, too.

As a psychotherapist, an essential part of my work is to check out whether my understanding of a client's experience, emotions and thoughts is accurate. I look for signs that suggest I'm not quite getting it, and then work to fill in what I'm missing.

This is more critical with Kara since the accident. At times she is less able to clearly articulate things and may blame herself if I don't understand. At one time she was willing to settle for my limited understanding. Lately she expects more and has learned to call me on it if I don't quite get it, usually in a letter. I have become vigilant about paying attention, not making assumptions, and clarifying every nuance. My patience has increased. In short, I have become attuned to greater subtlety.

The articles and experts on brain injury helped us both understand symptoms that, at times, seemed incomprehensible. We both drew comfort from knowing that much of what she was experiencing was a predictable, organic response to this type of injury.

I have also developed a great respect for what I *don't* know. I have learned to allow my lack of specialized expertise guide me and keep me from going too fast; to help me avoid making wrong assumptions and jumping to premature conclusions; and perhaps most important of all, to cause me to *truly* listen.

To Kara and others like her who have taught such lessons to people like me, a heartfelt "thank you."

Knowing that some readers of this book may be walking the same road Kara did, she and I each developed a list of recommendations to help choose a therapist.

Kara's list includes considerations specific to those who have experienced brain injury:

- Consider the hours and location a therapist is available. Look at what part of the day you can set aside and how that will affect the rest of your obligations. Often a session will leave you fatigued and that can, at the very least, diminish capacity to fulfill later requirements (kids, job . . .). At the very worst, it can be downright dangerous if you have to drive or care for small children after a draining session.

- The initial discussion should include the therapist's training and experience. Experience lends a therapist maturity, and a potentially broader understanding of your unique situation. It can help the therapist get past simple textbook approaches, and as a brain injury victim you might need that. Also, by having the therapist talk about experience, goals and philosophies, you have the opportunity to gauge how easily you can track his or her conversational quality (cadence, clarity, and precision).

- Ask them what they know about brain injury. Do they personally know of anyone who is brain injured? Do they understand the complexities of emotional damage after such an injury? Ask them what they imagine the residual effects from such an injury might be. You're looking for comprehension of and ability to relate to your condition.

- Different recovery stages involve different issues. Right after the injury I was dealing with denial and anger. Later stages brought problems with acceptance and adjustment. Ideally, you'll find a "therapist for all seasons." If not, different therapists for different stages might be needed.

- The therapist will need to know about and be able to deal with safety issues. Two that come to mind are that the patient might fall, or the patient might become angry. These, and many other contingencies, can provide taxing moments for both patient and therapist.

- It's possible that trying to select a therapist might be too exhausting during the early recovery process. You may

be overwhelmed with all the other treatments and pro-
cesses you're going through. If the idea of therapy is
overwhelming, maybe the time is just not right. In that
case, you might start the inner exploration yourself by
keeping a written journal.

- Researching and reference checking potential therapists
  is important.

- A therapist might not have the answers you seek, but just
  helping you to ask the right questions adds great value.

- If the issue of medication arises, it is vital that the therapist interact with the treating physician. Both sides need
  to know what the other is doing to effectively coordinate
  your treatment.

- Involve family and friends in your therapy, and make
  sure the therapist has an inclusive style that makes that
  possible.

- Don't look for magical overnight improvement. It may be
  months before you get any beneficial results.

- To get the most out of your therapy sessions, prepare
  written notes about what you want to cover. One thing
  we learn (even if we have a hard time remembering it) is
  that we can't count on our memories.

- If your case goes to court, there are legal/confidentiality
  issues to be dealt with. Your attorney can give you and
  your therapist important guidance on this.

My own list of recommendations is more general:

- Consider your goals and needs when you consider the
  qualities and qualifications of your therapist. It is like

choosing a physician. If you are selecting a surgeon, personality is of little relevance: expertise and technique are the critical criteria. Choosing a therapist is like choosing a family doctor: you want someone who is willing to really listen, and with whom you would feel comfortable talking about very private matters.

- Talk to others in therapy and find out what they like and don't like about their therapist. For example, I have a very nonlinear style. You can tell me a story from the middle, go back to the beginning, and weave in one or two other themes—and I will follow. My interviews have the same quality. I will follow whatever seems essential rather than force a chronology or order to the dialogue. Some people find this lack of formal structure annoying (or worse). Others find it suits them.

- Try to speak with the therapist before your first appointment. (Many of us make our own appointments, but at some clinics a receptionist handles this task.) Do not expect a lengthy conversation, but your first impression should give you a sense of the warmth of the therapist and help you feel welcomed.

- It's normal to be anxious about first seeing a therapist, but after the first session you should feel that the person was easy to talk to and paid attention to you. If after the third session you aren't feeling comfortable, find a new therapist.

- Remember: it is *your* therapy. You should feel part of a collaborative process. It should not feel as if something is being done *to* you.

- Your therapist should be interested in your unique experience, and in your view of what is happening within you and around you. It can be reassuring to hear that part of what you are going through is an expected—perhaps enduring—part of the injury, but that's not all there is to your story. For example, how do you handle unexplained anger? How do you and your family members cope with it?

- Your insurance may have some constraints on whom you can see and for how many sessions. Make sure you know what your policy says and don't squander your sessions with a therapist you don't like.

- Consider paying out of pocket rather than using your insurance if you can't find someone within your insurance plan who meets your needs. Many of us will adjust our fees, as processing insurance forms is time-consuming and expensive.

- Therapists are like clothing. Not everyone looks great in black or likes wearing it. Choose what suits you.

- It may take several tries to get it right. Don't stop looking until you find the right person for you.

—Virginia (Ginger) Keena, MA, LLP

Team Kara

Change is the prevailing constant in our lives. Kara Swanson speaks compellingly of change no one wants. The changes she documents in this painstaking journal are phenomenological nightmares, irritants and everything in between. They are interrupted career and life opportunities sealed off behind newly installed locks; the easy made difficult. As a rehabilitation counselor, it is my job to understand where there might be keys to release some of these locks. With passageways reopened, we can then identify opportunities and possible working identities.

In my early work with Kara, I learned how everything in her life had changed from a past she had loved. Her sense of stability, firmness under foot, was gone. An athlete, a manager whose workweek and pace might have doubled her 40-hour-per-week employees, she was suddenly unable to stand up and make the room around her behave as it should. She had been highly organized, capable of performing complex tasks. Now she struggled just to accomplish daily basics.

She described her anger and frustrations with great verbal eloquence—her broken furniture providing equally eloquent nonverbal communication. The sense of being strong, having stamina, being bright, being in control, having good friends, *being* a good friend, were all suddenly gone. No corner of her life escaped the simple, awful and final fact of change because of her head injury. Her challenge was to get back a vision of a "me," of her fundamental identity which had been terrifyingly lost in the accident.

During this process, it was my job to listen until Kara taught me how best to work with her. It was important that I hear the anguish—but discern it from despair. We needed to be alert to cues which would reveal the possibilities for healing and recovering her life.

I do this with my clients by listening closely, learning what people really care about. While every individual is unique, I have found over the years that the following guidelines are the most helpful for anyone rebuilding daily life after a severe disruption.

- **Know yourself.** Where are you strong? Where do you have trouble? Ask people you can trust and emphasize to them that their honesty helps more than it hurts.

- **Strengthen areas of weakness.** Therapies can help; make maximal use of them. Research. Experiment.

- **Organize and simplify.** Organize your thoughts, your workplace, the rooms you live in. Use one planner—only one—and use it for *everything*—business, social life, house and car maintenance, etc. Streamline your life, eliminating activities that take more than they give.

- **Don't waste energy—it's too precious.** Don't memorize anything that can be retrieved by turning a page or touching a keyboard. With a well-conceived, well-developed planner you can carry more information than you'll ever remember.

- **Protect your supports.** If you are lucky, there are people in your life who care about you. Their lives are changed, too. They are in a position to help. They provide comfort, but they can also tell you the truth when you need it or when they need it. Treat them with respect. Treat them well.

- **Remember what you care about.** How did you spend your time and money when your life was better? What interested you? Hobbies are more than just fun. If we look closely there, we usually find our hearts. We may also find some skill that can be translated to work.

- **What is your vocational identity?** Can you still perform elements of this work? Are there other jobs or interest areas where these skills have value? Explore widely. Be open to possibilities. (An excellent resource for anyone reevaluating vocation is the book *What Color Is Your Parachute?* by Richard Bolles, Ten Speed Press.)

- **Protect yourself.** Regardless of your positive feelings for those you care about, *you* are the most important person to your well-being and success. Be objective about the values and allegiances of those who promise to help you. Take care of yourself first. You can't help others without being strong yourself.

- **Operate with a plan.** Evaluate every challenge you face. Take time to prepare. The strategy you develop provides you an opportunity to grow stronger.

- **Always have a backup plan.** Some situations can become intolerable even with the best plans. If necessary, plan an avenue of escape. This is not failure; on the contrary, this is another strategy for success, another part of your game plan.

Kara may have lost her ability to play softball, but she certainly did not lose her understanding of the game or of sports. As a coach herself, she was grounded in the hallmarks of success in team sports. Concepts such as "discipline," "team play," "ground rules," "game plan" and "focus" were so close to her that they were ritual: only metaphors to some, but carrying real meaning for her. We see in this book how she evaluates and bonds with her therapists, her friends and all those in her support system. They're now her TEAM KARA.

This book traces the development of her new sense of "me." It's an identity markedly different from her pre-injury self. But it's a good identity, fit to meet the challenges she faces, built around abilities she still has or could get back. Yes, tracking words on a printed page might be difficult for her because of lingering neurological damage. But she can generate creative ideas, giving them life with a vibrant sense of language that is still very much alive and in fine health.

Does the emergence of a strong identity as a writer mean she will no longer be frustrated and sometimes angered by her problems with balance, physical strength and stamina? Certainly not. But it does mean she can use similar discipline and strategies to build her strength, improve her conditioning and physically stabilize herself, learning what is safe for her and what isn't.

I'll Carry the Fork! could as well have been titled *I'll Take Responsibility!* or *I Won't Be Beaten Down by This!* That resolve, fortified with a wonderfully insightful sense of humor and a game plan, is Kara's foundation for a strong identity, a "me" who can still compete. Kara has given us a blueprint for dealing with the damage done by brain injury—or *any* injury—recovering a life and building a future.

—*Robert Nettleman, MA, CRC, LPC*
Associate Chief of Clinical Services
Spectrum Rehabilitation Centers, Inc.

Team Kara

NOTES FROM AN ATTORNEY
SPECIALIZING IN BRAIN INJURY LITIGATION

I am a lawyer who specializes in representing traumatic brain injury survivors. That focus started many years ago. A 19-year-old woman who had suffered a concussion in a car crash came to my office with her mother. During the course of my interview, the young lady, whom I will call Mary, was able to answer questions and seemed perfectly fine to me. At one point in the meeting, Mary asked to use the restroom. While she was gone, her mother told me that since the crash, Mary was a different person: she had lost her job as a cashier in a restaurant, she seemed forgetful and she was irritable. She had not had these problems before.

After this information was confirmed in a later interview with Mary's sister, I must confess that as a fairly new lawyer, I did not know what to do. It was suggested to me that Mary had psychiatric problems, and I was fortunate enough to be able to refer Mary to a very prominent forensic psychiatrist for examination. The psychiatrist wrote a report saying that Mary had "organic brain dysfunction." As far as I knew at that stage in my life, the word "organic" referred to growing vegetables without fertilizer.

I made an appointment with the forensic psychiatrist, Dr. Emanuel Tanay. He spent four hours answering my questions. It was this conference which gave me my initial look into the world of traumatic brain injury and concussion, and the consequences they carried.

Since that time, I have been directly involved in litigation for hundreds of people surviving traumatic brain injury and have consulted with lawyers around the country in similar cases. This has involved intense research, attending many seminars and conferences, and spending hours upon hours with experts from such fields as psychiatry, biomechanical engineering, neuropsychology, vocational rehabilitation, life care planning and rehabilitation, and economics. I have represented persons surviving traumatic brain injury in a number of states, and have given over 200 invited lectures and presentations for various groups around the United States and Europe.

Several months ago, I received a call from a woman inviting me to speak at a seminar. She told me they were planning a presentation on how to *lose* a case involving traumatic brain injury—and they wanted to take advantage of my expertise! After a long, *long* pause, she began to apologize and I said, "No, that's OK, I am probably also an expert in losing these cases as well."

Although it sometimes seems like a well-kept secret, the incidence of brain injury in this country is ever increasing, and the price, in terms of pain, suffering, and lack of understanding, is astronomical. Brain injury is an insidious epidemic that knows no boundaries of race, religion, age or wealth. It is a most democratic injury: it can happen in the finest luxury car or an old pick-up truck; on the sprawling acreage of the finest mansion or the front porch of a house in the ghetto; to young or old. Even the finest education and the largest income are no guarantee of safety. The closed hand of brain injury can knock on any door, in any neighborhood, and always find someone home.

Even though we are now in the eighth year of the "decade of the brain," there are still far too many misconceptions, false notions and myths regarding traumatic brain injury (TBI). Here are some of the major ones:

- That a person has to be knocked out or in a coma to suffer a life-altering TBI.

- That a person needs to strike his or her head in order to have a life-altering TBI.

- That a normal skull X-ray, CT scan, neurological examination or MRI of the brain automatically means that there is not a life-altering TBI.

- That the person's problems are psychiatric and not the organic effects of TBI.

- That a brain injury described as "mild" or "minor" somehow means that the brain injury is not serious or significant (actually, the use of the words "mild" or "minor" is often very misleading in describing the consequences of a traumatic brain injury).

- That children easily bounce back from, and are unaffected by, mild to moderate TBI.

- That a child who does well in first or second grade following a TBI is completely cured without any long-term consequences.

- That a high postinjury IQ automatically means there has not been a life-altering TBI.

- That all TBIs are diagnosed in the hospital emergency room, or within the first month following the injury.

- That a person with a "mild" TBI should necessarily be able to work and earn money in competitive employment.

- That everybody gets better in 90 days.

Kara Swanson was very fortunate to have received the excellent medical care of Dr. Sharon L. Cini. This type of care, treatment and concern goes a long way toward dispelling myths and misconceptions. It should be commonplace in the world of mild to moderate TBI. Unfortunately, it is not.

Although some of my clients have been blessed with seven-figure verdicts and settlements in cases involving "mild" traumatic brain injury, every case is still like guerrilla warfare. That's because the defense lawyers and insurance companies start with the belief that all the myths mentioned above are true.

The coldness to injured people that defense lawyers and insurance companies sometimes display may stem from a lack of human understanding; or from ignorance; or, in some cases (I hate to say it) from mean-spiritedness; and in other cases, from a genuine belief that something invisible cannot be disabling. I have always considered that a part of my job in litigation was to *educate* defense lawyers and insurance companies about the realities of the injury and the case. Part of this education process happens during depositions of defense experts. Often it involves obtaining admissions that the various myths about TBI are untrue.

Over the years, I have been lectured by judges who have told me that people *should* get better from "mild" brain injury; and that if good lawyers can complete a jury trial involving a wrongful death in three days, why was I asking for a two-week trial for a "mild" brain injury case? And how could I expect anyone to believe there was a TBI when the CT scan was normal?

I have also listened to similar disparaging lectures from defense lawyers, insurance company representatives, facilitators and mediators. There are days when I get tremendously discouraged. Those are the days when I think it would be easier to specialize in broken legs. Then I could just hold up an X-ray. I wouldn't have to put up with the innuendo, or the insults about my clients being fakers, malingerers, having emotional problems, or that things from their past just finally "caught up with them"—coincidentally, on the day of the crash.

It is on those days of discouragement that my faith in God is often renewed and strengthened. Whether it's the Holy Spirit or something else, when I'm at the low point, something always happens to get me energized and back on track. It might be a letter from a client, or even a nonclient, thanking me for understanding; perhaps a letter from someone who has read one of my articles; or a card from a secretary in my office. It makes me realize again why I do what I do.

In one of my "down" moments, I got a much-needed lift from my friend Sharon Barefoot, who spent many years as the president of the Michigan Head Injury Alliance, then served with distinction on the board of directors of the National Head Injury Foundation (now Brain Injury Association). She told me that she thought I was one of those whom God had chosen to fight for, and speak on behalf of, those who could not fight for or speak for themselves. Because of my strong spiritual beliefs, I have always thought this was the greatest compliment or honor I could receive.

I have also been privileged to have the opportunity to work with, and learn from, some of the world's foremost experts on issues related to TBI and its consequences. I am grateful that these incredibly busy people have spent hours answering my questions, providing me with education that I can place in the service of injured persons in need of help.

We live in a society where information about medicine, injuries and recovery rates is widely known. For example, if someone breaks a leg, the surgical insertion of a plate and six screws will cause that person to be out of action for six to nine months or so. The casting, scarring and obvious disability make it unnecessary for the injured person to explain why he or she can't walk or run so well at the moment.

Or, if someone has a heart attack, even untrained lay people know it will be a while before the victim will be returning to work or rejoining his golf foursome. News of the heart attack makes it unnecessary for the victim to have to explain that he now has some limitations.

None of this is true about the outcome of traumatic brain injury—whether mild, moderate, or severe—because it is so unpredictable. With many injuries or conditions, the doctor can confidently predict the limitations. A torn knee ligament means no skiing. Simple. Traumatic brain injury is more subtle. The symptoms may be as elusive as difficulty understanding music or multiple conversations at a party. They may be impossible to clearly explain to family members, friends and former co-workers.

Far too many physicians conduct their practice without knowing the information contained in the following quote from the book *Mild Head Injury* by Levin, Eisenberg and Benton (pp. 3–4):

> Post concussion syndrome is generally understood to refer to a condition in which a person who has sustained a concussion complains of a variety of somatic, cognitive, emotional, motor, or sensory disabilities which he or she ascribes to the concussion. At the same time, convincing historical and clinical evidence of significant brain injury cannot be elicited. The typical history indicates that at the time of the accident and shortly thereafter, the person was comatose for only a brief period if at all, and showed practically no retrograde amnesia and very little posttraumatic amnesia. ...Weeks or months after the accident, the patient will voice one or more complaints which, in their totality, have come to be called the posttraumatic symptom-complex or syndrome. Prominent features of the syndrome include headache, impairment in attention and concentration, poor memory, depression and emotional instability, lowered tolerance of frustration, sleep disturbances, loss of sexual drive, and intolerance to alcohol. The net effect of these impairments often (but by no means always) is to render the person signifi-

cantly handicapped from a social and economic standpoint. However, at this time, clinical examination discloses very little cognitive, motor, or sensory deficit that can be reasonably ascribed to brain injury, and, in the opinion of the examining physician, the findings are essentially negative. Thus there is a striking discrepancy between the presumably "subjective" complaints of the patient and the presumably "objective" findings of the physician; this almost inevitably leads to an uncomfortable state of cognitive dissonance in both parties and sometimes to open conflict between them.
...

Early clinicians were also well aware that apparently mild head injuries, as indicated by the history, could have the most serious long-term consequences.

The following description of the life of a person surviving TBI is particularly poignant for those who have not received the benefit of a diagnosis. It should be read and reread by anyone trying to gain some basic understanding of this area. In her book, *Neuropsychological Assessment, Second Edition*, Dr. Muriel D. Lezak writes (pp. 10–11):

Most people who sustain brain injury experience changes in their intellectual and emotional functioning, but because they are on the inside, so to speak, they may have difficulty appreciating how their behavior has changed and what about them is still the same. These misperceptions tend to heighten what mental confusion may already be present as a result of altered patterns of neural activity.

Distrust of their experiences, particularly their memory and perceptions, is another problem shared by many brain damaged persons, probably as a result of even very slight disruptions and alterations of the exceedingly complex neural pathways that mediate the intellectual function. This distrust seems to arise from the feelings of strangeness and confusion accompanying previously familiar habits, thoughts, and sensations that are now experienced differently.

. . . Even quite subtle deficits in motivation, in abilities to plan, organize, and carry out activities, and in self-monitoring can compromise a patient's capacity to earn a living and may render him socially dependent as well. Moreover, many brain damaged patients no longer fit easily into family life as their irritability, self-centeredness, impulsivity, or apathy create awesome emotional burdens on family members, generate conflicts between family members and with the patient, and strain family ties, often beyond endurance.

In her article entitled "Subtle Sequelae of Brain Damage, Perplexity, Distractability, and Fatigue," Dr. Lezak writes:

The patient is in the position of someone whose clock has just struck 13. Not only does he know

the clock is wrong, but the error casts doubt on
all that follows.

Think about the last time your watch started to lose a few
minutes every day. By the end of every week, if uncorrected,
the watch would be 20 or 30 minutes more behind. Even
though physically it might still be a good-looking, expensive
watch, statistically still 99 percent effective, most of us
would get a new watch. But persons surviving TBI do not
have the luxury of buying a new part. They must adjust to
figuring out what time it is with a slightly defective watch.

When we think about long-term consequences of TBI, the
following quote from Dr. Dorothy Gronwall, in her article
entitled "Cumulative and Persisting Effects of Concussion
on Attention and Cognition," informs us:

> After mild head injury, patients have difficulty
> in all areas that require them to analyze more
> items of information than they can handle
> simultaneously. They present as slow because it
> takes longer for smaller than normal chunks of
> information to be processed. They present as
> distractible because they do not have the spare
> capacity to monitor irrelevant stimuli at the
> same time as they are attending to the relevant
> stimulus. They present as forgetful because
> while they are concentrating on point A, they
> do not have the processing space to think about
> point B simultaneously. They present as inat-
> tentive because when the amount of informa-
> tion that they are given exceeds their capacities,
> they cannot take it all in.

...Even those patients who appear to have made a full functional recovery, who record normal scores on all neuropsychological tests, and who have returned to their pre-injury social and work life, may demonstrate persistent impairment when subjected to another stress. ...We are all vulnerable to stress and tension in our work and family lives, but mild head injury patients continue to have an extra vulnerability. There is no evidence to show that this vulnerability decreases over time since injury.

At p. 36 of *Neuropsychological Assessment—Second Edition,* Dr. Muriel D. Lezak states:

Many persons suffer profound personality changes following brain injury, or concomitant with brain disease, which seems not so much a direct product of their illness as a reaction to their experience of loss, chronic frustration, and radical changes in lifestyle. As a result, depression is probably the most common single characteristic of brain damaged patients, generally with pervasive anxiety following closely behind. ...For the most part, the personality changes, emotional distress and behavior problems of a brain damaged patient are the product of extremely complex interactions involving neurological disabilities, present social demands, previously established behavioral patterns and ongoing reaction to all of these.

In an article entitled "Disability Caused by Minor Head Injury," *Neurosurgery*, Vol. 9, No. 3, p. 221 (1981), Rimel, Giordani, Barth, Boll and Jane discussed a study of some 538 patients having sustained minor head trauma with loss of consciousness of 20 minutes or less, and with a Glasgow Coma Scale of 13 to 15. As stated at p. 226:

> The most important finding from this study is the large number of patients with minor head injury who were experiencing difficulties with their lives three months after injury. ...More than one-half of the patients complained of memory deficits ...one-third of our patients who were gainfully employed before injury were unemployed three months later. ...Most patients scored lower than their expected norms on the neuropsychological battery, with the principal problems being cognitive deficits in the spheres of attention and concentration, memory and judgment. ...One of the most important questions raised by this study was the incidence and importance of organic brain damage in patients who are rendered unconscious briefly by a blow to the head. The neurological examination did not contribute much to the solution of this question. Aside from the score on the Glasgow Coma Scale, only a very small number of patients had a slightly abnormal neurological examination on admission, all were normal at discharge, and very few patients had an abnormality at follow up and EEG compatible with that diagnosis.

At p. 221 of this study is this statement:

> Also, neuronal loss has been found during post-mortem examination of patients in whom the only known head injury was a concussion and in whom there was no obvious clinical evidence of brain damage.

This article then goes on to this very powerful and poignant conclusion at p. 227:

> The findings of this study provide evidence for a sequence of events after minor head injury that has been suggested by other investigators. According to our hypothesis, the head injury in many of these patients is much more significant than was assumed in the past. The patient sustained organic brain damage that causes problems in attention, concentration, memory and judgment. For the most part they recognize these deficits and are disturbed by them. The disturbance is all the greater because the patients were assured at discharge that the injury was inconsequential and that therefore recovery should be immediate and complete. Neither the patients nor their families understand why they are continuing to have so much difficulty, and the harder the patients try, the more anxious and frustrated they become. In time the patients may become incapacitated by the psychological responses to their injuries

even though the organic defects may have largely disappeared.

It is also well known and recognized that what appear to be late-developing cognitive, emotional, behavioral and other problems in children may be the consequence of a pediatric traumatic brain injury. In his book, *Closed Head Injury: A Clinical Sourcebook*, p. 174, Dr. Peter G. Bernad writes:

> There is a misunderstanding among health care professionals about the effects of mild to moderate head injury in children. A common assumption prevails that infants who are brain injured recover more quickly and completely than adults. However, there is mounting evidence that infants tolerate head injury less well than any other age group. Beyond infancy, the relationship between age and recovery is less clear. The medical data are frequently conflicting. There is a growing body of evidence indicating that children experience more pervasive long term cognitive and behavioral sequelae than had been previously recognized. ...The theory of the "plasticity" of the child's brain is unfounded. Children experience significant problems after mild to moderate head injury, including post-concussive syndrome.

When thinking about pediatric brain injury, think about the example of a seven-year-old second grader, an all-A student, who suffers a moderate traumatic brain injury in May, and is out of school for the rest of the semester. In September, A and B report cards continue, which adds to the notion that there has been a full recovery from the TBI. As the child gets to the fifth, sixth and seventh grades, school becomes much more difficult, grades are more like Cs and Ds, the child becomes frustrated, behavioral problems develop, the child ends up in trouble, and no one remembers the TBI. Remember, second and third grade are not that intellectually challenging, and the parts of the child's brain that were injured and damaged may not have been called upon until the more complex demands in the fifth, sixth and seventh grades.

Consider that a five-foot barrel has a gaping hole at the four-foot mark. So long as there is only one foot of water in the barrel, it performs just fine; the barrel's vulnerability at the four-foot mark has not been challenged. As water goes to the two- and three-foot mark, the barrel still functions with no problem. But at the four-foot mark, the barrel starts leaking. If it took three years for the water to go from the one-foot to the four-foot mark, finally exposing the damaged area, some might not realize that the problem had been there all along. They might assume it developed only when the water got to the four-foot mark, rather than years before. In a much more complex sense, this type of thinking applies to the consequences of pediatric TBI.

The reality is that some children and teenagers are condemned to a lifetime of silent screaming, suffering, frustration and failure because no one has considered that their problems may be related to a TBI—and are not their fault.

I recently saw a cartoon in which a young lawyer was joking that while he had lost a case, he had gained a lot of experience. I didn't find this very funny. In our justice system, a person surviving injuries has only one opportunity *per life-*

time to bring a case to trial for those injuries. If he or she is represented by an attorney who is inexperienced, unprepared, uncommitted or otherwise incompetent, the injured person will suffer the double punishment of being injured in the first place, then not receiving appropriate compensation.

There is a somewhat idealistic notion in our society that "right makes might." This may be true in some settings, but it absolutely does not apply in the legal arena. If an attorney does not know what he or she is doing, or does not understand the injury, or does not understand how to prove the existence and extent of the injury, then no matter how compelling, truthful and just the case may be, that attorney's client may end up with nothing.

Many years ago, there were few lawyers who would take on cases involving mild to moderate TBI. In fact, in my early days, I was sometimes the sixth or eighth lawyer that a person or family would consult in trying to obtain legal representation. Now, things have changed. Multimillion dollar verdicts and settlements involving "mild" TBI have been achieved and publicized. This has caused a tremendous proliferation of attorneys attending seminars, then representing themselves as competent and experienced in handling these cases.

Perceiving that there is quick money to be made in representing persons with TBI, many of these law firms run elaborate television, magazine and newspaper ads. Some of these same lawyers then call me literally on Friday afternoon, seeking advice and guidance about what to do in a brain injury case they are bringing to trial on Monday. Unfortunately, attending one or two seminars does not make a lawyer competent or experienced. Just as a person surviving TBI needs specialized medical care, treatment and therapy, so also does he or she need specialized legal representation.

Because contingent fee agreements are prevalent throughout the United States, every person can afford to hire the best and most qualified lawyer to handle an injury case. Regardless of social, educational or economic background, anyone with a legal claim involving injury or death can walk into the finest and fanciest law firm. They will receive courteous, respectful and experienced assistance because of the contingent fee agreement. Injured people need not settle for the second best lawyer, or the second most experienced lawyer. And in making the selection, the person should remember: *this may very well represent the one and only opportunity they will have to seek compensation for the entire lifetime of suffering caused by the negligence of someone else.*

As consumers, we all know how to evaluate and purchase things like cars, refrigerators and houses. But when it comes to hiring professionals like lawyers, we are often at a loss. The purpose of this section is to empower and assist traumatic brain injury survivors, and their families, in selecting and hiring the most qualified attorney possible.

I suggest that at the initial interview with an attorney, a person use the guideline below to question the attorney about education, experience and competence in handling cases similar to the one being presented. At the conclusion of the interview, the attorney should be asked to sign the form, acknowledging that the answers given are true. If the attorney will not sign it, run, don't walk, to the nearest exit. The questions that must be answered, and my recommendations for what constitutes acceptable answers, are as follows:

1. Over the past 3 years, how many cases similar to mine have you been involved with as the principal attorney? *(If the answer is fewer than 10, you should be polite but leave.)*

---

2. Over the past 5 years, in how many cases have you actually gone to trial as the lead lawyer and received a jury verdict representing injuries similar to mine? What have the verdicts been? *(If the answer is fewer than 5 trials, and/or if 3 or more were losses, be polite but leave.)*

---

3. What percentage of your practice of law is devoted to cases and injuries similar to mine? *(If the answer is less than 75 percent, be polite but leave.)*

---

4. What were the settlements or verdicts for the last 10 cases you handled involving injuries similar to mine? *(If the answer is that more than 5 were under $100,000, be polite but leave.)*

---

5. How many seminars or conferences have you attended over the past 2 years involving presentations on injuries similar to mine? *(If the answer is fewer than 5, be polite but leave.)*

---

6. How many articles have you written over the past 3 years involving any aspect of injury similar to mine? *(If the answer is fewer than 5, be polite but leave. Writing articles is not always critical to a lawyer's competence and experience, but not having published some in this specialized area may be a warning sign.)*

_____

_____

7. Over the last 3 years, how many lectures have you been invited to give on issues related to injuries similar to mine? *(If the answer is 10 or fewer, it might be a good idea to be polite but leave.)*

_____

_____

8. Please list 3 textbooks you own and refer to when discussing or reviewing information on injuries similar to mine. *(Make sure they produce the textbooks, and make sure they look somewhat worn or well read.)*

_____

_____

9. If necessary, would you and your law firm be able and willing to spend as much as $75,000 in advance to investigate, prepare and present my case, as a part of the contingent fee arrangement? *(Depending upon the cause of the injuries, the nature and extent of the injuries and the ability to collect from potential defendants, this is a very important question. It is not uncommon for law firms to spend over $100,000 putting the case together. If you are dealing with a lawyer who is not a named partner, that lawyer may not have the fiscal authority to commit his firm to this level of*

expenditure. If you cannot get a commitment in this regard, be polite but leave.)

---

10. What experts do you expect to hire to assist you with the analysis and presentation of my case? *(If the attorney seems at a loss to understand or discuss any of these potential experts, be polite but leave.)*

    • Neuropsychologists:

    • Forensic psychiatrists:

    • Accident reconstruction experts:

    • Vocational economic analysts:

    • Forensic economists:

    • Biomechanical engineers:

    • Life and care planning specialists:

    Are there any other experts you believe would be helpful in presenting my case?

(SIGNATURE OF ATTORNEY)

❧

To understand the life of people surviving traumatic brain injury, you have to spend time with them. You must get up close and personal to appreciate the subtle problems. I depend on that "face time" with my clients to stoke the fire in my soul for trial and representation.

I have had lunch with clients who insisted on it being their treat, but when the bill came, they simply could not figure out whether to give a $20 bill, a $50 bill or some other bill for a $17 check. I have seen numerous examples of memory lapses, such as the lady who wanted a barbecued steak, went to the store to buy the steak, returned home, put it on the grill in the backyard—and was absolutely astounded 30 minutes later to see firemen in her yard putting out the fire in the barbecue.

Years ago, during the third week of a jury trial, the plaintiff came to testify. I had been working on her case for two years. Yet when she saw me that day, she said "I swear you look familiar. I feel like I know you from somewhere!" She just could not make the connection that I was her lawyer. I know I don't make much of an impression physically, but I thought my diminutive stature, thinning hair and high-pitched voice might have made *some* mark on this woman's mind over two years! I know she was not faking the lack of recognition (although, I must confess, I have occasionally run into people who *did* pretend not to know me. I try not to take it personally).

When I see these dramatic and heartbreaking effects of clients' injuries, it motivates me to do everything I can to get them the compensation they deserve.

❧

Many years ago, the late Dr. Martin Luther King, Jr., offered the following words of eternal truth. They seem particularly meaningful for persons experiencing the consequences of brain injury:

> May you never forget that through it all,
> God walks with you.
> Never forget that God is able to lift you
> From the fatigue of despair to the buoyancy of hope,
> And transform dark and desolate valleys
> Into sunlit paths of inner peace.

My involvement with parents and families taking care of loved ones surviving brain injury has been a tremendous source of personal inspiration, energy and humility. In all of this, there is a simple, straightforward, common thread: *we need each other.* We must all work together to share, educate, love, understand and grow, so that the plight of persons surviving brain injury may be made just a little easier to bear. The more we share the load, the less weight each of us has to carry.

In the faces and dedication of those persons who support injury survivors, I have seen the true spirit of the words from Matthew 25:35-36. I dedicate this biblical paraphrase to you: "…I had a brain injury, and you tried to help." In that same spirit, Kara Swanson looks up from her injury and says "How can I help others?" I am honored that I was asked to contribute to her book.

May God bless all of you with the gifts of courage, determination and hope.

—*Charles N. (Nick) Simkins, Esq.*
Northville, Michigan

Ms. Swanson is an experienced, inspirational, and informative speaker. To arrange to have Ms. Swanson speak to your group, please contact Rising Star Press.

 Rising Star Press
Quality Books that Inform and Inspire

P.O. Box 66378
Scotts Valley, CA 95067-6378
Phone 888-777-2207
Fax 831-461-0445
e-mail: editor@risingstarpress.com

Visit us on the Internet at www.RisingStarPress.com

This book was designed with the help of the author for easy readability by persons who have experienced brain injury. We welcome your comments.

Notes

Notes

Notes

Notes

Notes

Keep this form and your insurance card with you at all times.

Name: . . . . Phone: . . . .

Address: . . . .

Height: . . . . Weight: . . . . Birth date: . . . .

Wear glasses (circle one):   Y   N

Identifying marks, dental plates, artificial limbs, etc.: . . . .

. . . .

Current medications (include dosages): . . . .

. . . .

Challenges/symptoms that are normal for me: . . . .

. . . .

Primary care physician: . . . . Phone: . . . .

   Location of records on file: . . . .

Emergency contacts:

   Name . . . . Phone: . . . .

      Relation to patient: . . . .

   Name . . . . Phone: . . . .

      Relation to patient: . . . .

Medical history (applicable medical history, allergies, incidences, etc.):

. . . .

. . . .

Organ donor (circle one):   Y   N   Tissue donor (circle one):   Y   N

Religious affiliation: . . . .

Other: . . . .

Signature: . . . . Date: . . . .